EXERCISES
FOR
SCIATICA

EXERCISES

FOR

SCIATICA

A Simple and Effective
Self-Care Program for Pain Relief
and the Treatment of Sciatica

WILLIAM SMITH, MS, CSCS, MEPD
WAZIM BUKSH, MD, MPH

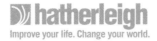

Improve your life. Change your world.

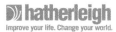
Improve your life. Change your world.

Hatherleigh Press is committed to preserving and protecting the natural resources of the earth. Environmentally responsible and sustainable practices are embraced within the company's mission statement.

Visit us at www.hatherleighpress.com and register online for free offers, discounts, special events, and more.

Exercises for Sciatica
Text copyright © 2020 William Smith and Wazim Buksh, MD, MPH

Library of Congress Cataloging-in-Publication Data is available upon request.
ISBN: 978-1-57826-788-0

Cover and Interior Design by Courtney Wade

Printed in the United States
10 9 8 7 6 5 4 3 2 1

Your health starts here! Workouts, nutrition, motivation, community . . . everything you need to build a better body from the inside out!

Visit us at www.getfitnow.com for videos, workouts, nutrition, recipes, community tips, and more!

Consult your physician before beginning any exercise program. The author and publisher of this book and workout disclaim any liability, personal or professional, resulting from the misapplication of any of the following procedures described in this publication.

CONTENTS

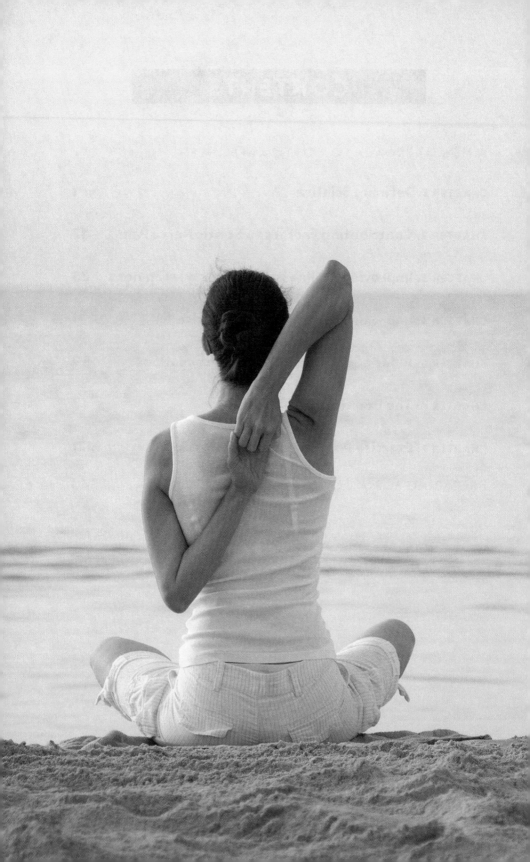

A New Approach to Sciatica Wellness

Here's a fun fact for you: the Centers for Disease Control (CDC) reports that Americans are sitting an average of 13 hours a day and sleeping an average of 8 hours, resulting in a sedentary lifestyle of **around 21 hours a day.**

The average American spends nearly half their day staring at a screen. A new audience report put out by the Nielsen Company reveals that adults in the United States devoted about 10 hours and 39 minutes each day to consuming media during the first quarter of 2019. This figure includes the time we spend—each and every day—using our tablets, smartphones, personal computers, televisions, and multimedia devices.

Is it any surprise that back pain symptoms are on the rise?

Of course, it's not all our own faults. Every day, we face life's unrelenting grind—the rigors of commuting to work, only to be figuratively chained to our desks for hours on end. For those eight hours (or more) we become "habitual sitters", as the same technology that has revolutionized the world creates a society of stagnation.

This lack of daily movement has led to rampant obesity, and a society full of individuals who have developed muscular imbalances and flexibility issues to their unhealthy lifestyle. Each day, they are made to deal with the ultimate consequence of these issues: chronic low back pain.

And it's not as though we can just "take it easy" and things will mend on their own. With every step we take, we subject our bodies to physical force that travels up from our feet and leads up to our spine, where various neural structures (our body's "electrical wiring") are housed—including the sciatic nerve, a large nerve that connects from the lower half of our spine to our lower legs. In combination with the imbalances caused by our sedentary lifestyles, the ground reaction forces from a single step transferred up this chain converge, placing pressure on our wiring and creating new and worsening pain.

Chronic low back pain and sciatica affect millions of Americans each year, with severity ranging from simply nagging to truly debilitating. Often multifactorial in nature, the pain can permeate to all aspects of an individual's life, leading to functional disability and crippling mental distress.

Fortunately, there's a fix. By incorporating more physical activity into your daily routine (even if it doesn't completely meet the recent government recommendations of 150 minutes of moderate to vigorous exercise a week), you can help offset some of the negative health effects of sitting for long periods of time.

Exercises for Sciatica was designed to provide a complete workout program and lifestyle guide for those suffering from low back pain and sciatica. Taking as its two primary focuses strengthening muscles and relieving pain, it addresses sciatic pain from a broad spectrum, bio-psycho-social perspective. We've chosen to tackle this pain by examining how it is influenced by physical strain and exacerbated by negative mental and emotional states, such as depression. In so doing, we provide a pragmatic approach to identifying causative elements and personal risk factors, and finding tangible solutions for symptom relief.

More than anything, sciatica is a condition brought about by an unhealthy lifestyle. Rather than resort to expensive, potentially addictive painkillers and prescription medication, we can choose to view this as a wake-up call to become more active and live a healthier, happier life.

Our goal is to empower you not only to identify the negative health factors in your routine but to find reliable, cost-effective strategies to both reverse symptoms and prevent future instances of sciatic pain. To that end, we've created an exercise program which has little to no cost, much of which requires no equipment beyond your own body. Using the same multidisciplinary approach employed by personal trainers, we then move beyond symptom relief and progress to true rehabilitation, restoring you to a functional state of well-being.

In this book, you will find information about the common causes of sciatica and its side effects, along with practical tips for managing symptoms and improving your quality of life. You will also find a complete exercise list and workout program, tailored to help strengthen those muscles which support the spine and increase circulation to the discs of the spine to relieve pressure on the sciatic nerve and reduce pain. These, along with other benefits, are all reasons why it is so important to include an exercise program as part of your complete approach to treating sciatica.

Sciatic pain is a state of aggravation and irritation that penetrates every aspect of wellness. While not all cases of sciatica are preventable, the simplest and most common-sense healthy lifestyle choices can greatly reduce your chances of developing it, keeping you active and pain-free. Together, let's resolve to learn how best to *respond* to this pain, rather than *react* to it.

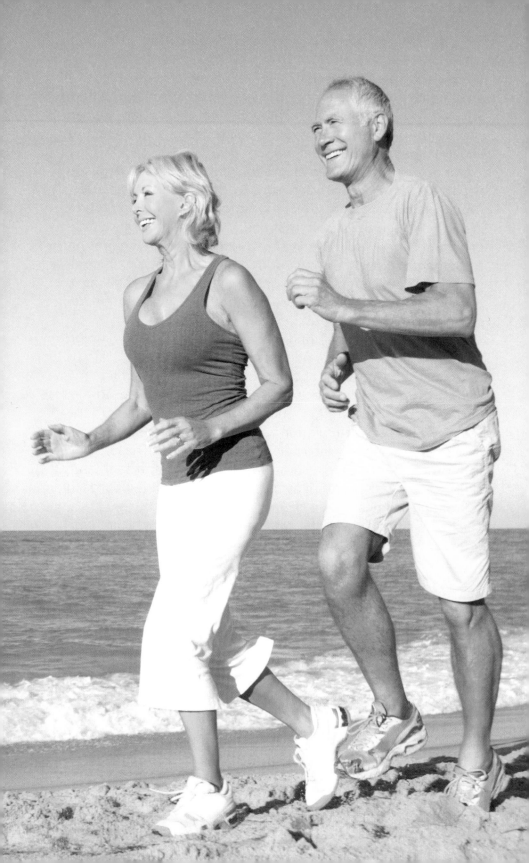

CHAPTER 1

Defining Sciatica

Back pain is one of the most common reasons that people go to see their doctors. Whether it is acute pain that develops suddenly or chronic pain that lingers for months, adults will often report having at least one day of back pain roughly every three months. Back pain—specifically pain related to the sciatic nerve, a long nerve pathway which runs from your lower back, through your hips and buttocks and down each leg—can seriously hamper mobility, disrupt sleep, and even take a psychological toll on someone during the days, weeks, or even months that their pain persists.

Thankfully, while the pain caused by sciatica is undoubtedly disruptive to a person's daily life, there are certain healthy choices and lifestyle changes anyone can make to help prevent the onset of back pain, control its severity, and reduce (or possibly even completely avoid) sciatic nerve pain. (While there *are* surgical options for the treatment of chronic sciatica, most cases of sciatica will subside with time. It is important to bear in mind that sciatica is a *symptom* of a medical problem; it is not a medical condition on its own.)

Of course, it is important for all people to develop good habits, such as maintaining a nutritious diet and remaining physically active. However, it is *especially* important for people who suffer from back pain to make healthy choices that can help them manage their sciatica for improved, long-term spinal health.

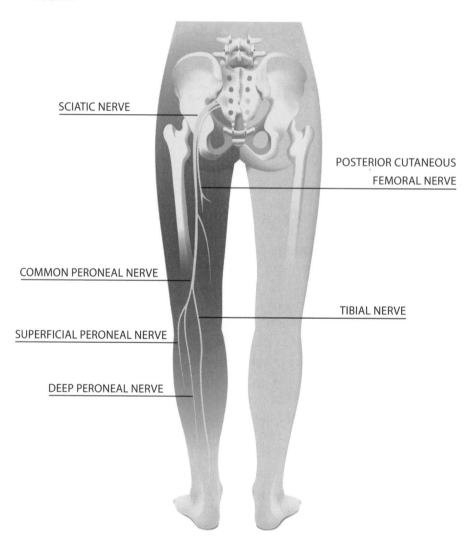

SCIATIC NERVE

POSTERIOR CUTANEOUS
FEMORAL NERVE

COMMON PERONEAL NERVE

TIBIAL NERVE

SUPERFICIAL PERONEAL NERVE

DEEP PERONEAL NERVE

A QUICK ANATOMY LESSON

It is often difficult to pinpoint the cause of back pain because the back itself is complex, and pain can radiate from damage or injury to any of the various bones, nerves, muscles, and ligaments that make up the back. So, before we can understand sciatica, we first have to understand the anatomy of the spine and its relationship to the sciatic nerve.

The spine is made up of a column of small bones called **vertebrae** that support the upper body. The **lumbar section** of the spine (which is where the pain of sciatica originates from) is found in the lower back and encompasses the five lowest—and largest—vertebrae, which support most of the body's weight and therefore come under the most stress. In between each of the vertebrae of the spinal column are **intervertebral discs,** which act as small cushions full of a gel-like substance called **nucleus pulposus.**

The **sciatic nerve,** the longest and widest nerve in the human body, runs from each side of the lower spine, or lumbar region, through the pelvis, into each buttock and down the length of the leg. The sciatic nerve acts as a pathway connecting the spinal cord with the muscles of the leg and foot. Pain that radiates along this nerve can be excruciating and debilitating for many patients.

Located in front of the piriformis muscle, the sciatic nerve is formed by many nerves that leave the lower spine and are joined into one nerve by a sheath of connective tissue, the most abundant substance in the human body. Among the nerves that make up the sciatic nerve are the lowest two nerves that exit from the lower spine (identified as L4 and L5) and the first three sacral nerves (identified as S1, S2 and S3).

Sciatica refers to any pain that radiates from the lower back or hip, down through the thigh and leg, and which is caused by an irritation of the sciatic nerve. When this nerve is constricted or the roots of the nerves are irritated, it can result in pain that begins in the lower back and often runs down the thigh, causing discomfort and numbness all the way down into the foot and toes. Sciatic pain can range in frequency and severity from sporadic and dull, to persistent and incapacitating. For more information and to gain a better understanding of human anatomy, we recommend the resources of both Tom Myers' Anatomy Trains and Gil Hedley's The Integral Anatomy series.

CAUSES OF SCIATICA

It's important to reiterate that sciatica itself is not a condition; rather, it is a symptom. Often, there is no one particular event that triggers sciatic nerve pain—compression of the nerve can develop simply because of general wear and tear over time. The location and severity of sciatica symptoms also varies depending on which part or parts of the nerve roots are affected.

Spinal Hernia

As we age, the spinal vertebrae weaken and are more suscep-tible to injury. Usually, sciatic pain is the result of a herniated or displaced disc that presses against the nerve root. A disc becomes **herniated** when it ruptures and the gel within it (the nucleus pulposus) pushes outward. While deteriorating and damaged discs are not uncommon, especially as we age, not ev-eryone with damaged discs will experience back pain. But when the gel from inside the disc extends out far enough to press against the sciatic nerve root, *that* is when you are most likely to experience pain.

Spinal Stenosis

While disc herniation is one of the most common causes of sci-atica, it is not the only cause. **Spinal stenosis** is another com-monly occurring condition that can lead to sciatica. Over time, a weakening of spinal vertebrae results in a narrowing of the spinal canal or a narrowing of the openings where nerves leave the spinal column. As a result, the spinal nerve roots that form the base of the sciatic nerve can become pinched. Spinal steno-sis is fairly common in adults over the age of 65.

Piriformis Syndrome

Another potential cause of sciatic nerve pain is **piriformis syn-drome.** The piriformis is a small muscle that is located in the buttock region. This flat, pyramid-shaped muscle connects to the upper surface of the femur and assists in stabilizing the femoral head and in rotating the hip. When that muscle contracts, it can compress the nearby sciatic nerve, which runs vertically beneath the muscle. In some people, the sciatic nerve can actually run right through the piriformis muscle. As a result, people can feel pain and numbness in the buttocks, hips, and legs due to spasms of the piriformis.

Injury

While most cases of sciatica can be attributed to the natural weakening and deterioration of the spine that comes with aging, another potential cause of sciatica pain is **injury.** Due to its location in the lower back, the sciatic nerve is susceptible to injuries caused by high-impact sports and activities like running on concrete, accidents such as a slip or a fall, or trauma that might be sustained during a car crash. Any number of incidents might cause the spine to move out of alignment and aggravate the sciatic nerve.

SCIATICA AND PREGNANCY

A population frequently at-risk for experiencing sciatica is pregnant women. Sometimes, the sciatic nerve can become pinched between the head of the fetus and the pelvic wall, resulting in pain and numbness through the buttocks and legs. Sciatica during pregnancy can also be attributed to muscle pain and unstable joints that result from increased hormones and the baby's weight.

Tumors

It is important to note that **tumors** may also cause sciatica, though this condition tends to be rare. If tumors form in the spinal region, they can put pressure on the nerve roots. You should always consult your doctor if you are concerned about pain.

DIAGNOSING SCIATICA

During a physical exam, your doctor may check your muscle strength and reflexes. For example, you may be asked to walk on your toes or heels, rise from a squatting position and, while lying on your back, lift your legs one at a time. Pain that results from sciatica will usually worsen during these activities.

Imaging Tests

Many people have herniated discs or bone spurs that will show up on X-rays and other imaging tests, but show no symptoms. Doctors don't typically order these types of tests unless your pain is severe, or it doesn't improve within a few weeks. Below is an overview of imaging tests that are commonly ordered to provide a more detailed perspective on sciatica patients. Your primary care provider will likely perform some manual testing before referring you to a specialist (such as an orthopedist, physiatrist (rehabilitation), or sports medicine trained internist) for further screening.

X-ray. An X-ray of your spine may reveal an overgrowth of bone called a bone spur that may be pressing on a nerve.

CT scan. Also called CAT scans, these are specialized X-ray tests performed to produce a cross-sectional image of the body, thereby providing doctors with more information to work from. Often times, a contrast dye will injected into your spinal canal before a CT scan in a procedure called a CT myelogram. The dye circulates around the spinal cord and spinal nerves and shows up more clearly on the final scan, making diagnosis more accurate.

MRI. An MRI (magnetic resonance imaging) scan produces detailed images of bone and soft tissues—such as herniated discs—by using a powerful magnet and radio waves to produce cross-sectional images of your back. This test requires you to lie on a table that moves into the MRI machine itself.

Electromyography (EMG). This test can show nerve compression caused by herniated discs or a narrowing of your spinal canal (called spinal stenosis) by measuring the muscles' response to electrical impulses.

In the next section, you will find some common symptoms and side effects of sciatica, along with practical suggestions for improving one's health. These have been designed specifically for those living with sciatic pain, but it is important to remember that sciatica does not affect everyone the same way, and that symptoms, signs, and severity will vary from person to person.

COMMON SYMPTOMS OF SCIATICA

Leg Pain

The primary symptom of sciatica is pain, concentrated in one of the lower extremities. Generally, sciatica affects only one side of the lower body, with pain being felt more acutely in the leg than in the lower back. Sciatic pain radiates from the lower portion of the spine, through the buttocks, down the thigh and through the leg, along the pathway of the sciatic nerve. The location and intensity of the pain will vary, depending on what portion of the sciatic nerve root is irritated.

Patients suffering from sciatica often report constant pain ranging from a dull ache to a sharp and shooting pain that leads to difficulties in standing or walking. You may also find that your pain increases when you attempt to change positions from lying down to sitting, or from sitting to standing. Your pain may also intensify during sudden movements, such as sneezing or coughing.

Depending on the cause of your sciatica, certain types of movement may elicit more pain than others. For example, if your pain increases when bending backwards or walking longer distances (50+ yards), this may be an indication that spinal stenosis is the source of your sciatic nerve pain. Conversely, if you experience increased levels of pain when bending forwards, this may indicate a herniated disc. Pay attention to the movements and activities that exacerbate your pain, so that you can accurately report your symptoms to your doctor.

TIPS FOR RELIEVING PAIN

Stay active. While bed rest might be tempting, it can actually make your pain last longer. It is important to try to maintain a normal activity level. Limit activities that cause excessive stretching or straining during the course of your day.

Take short breaks. Rest periodically throughout your day, as you normally would.

Avoid intense exercise. This includes any strenuous physical activity (particularly heavy lifting) during periods of back and leg pain.

Consider using an aid. A support such as a back brace or belt can provide some relief from sciatic pain, but should only be used temporarily, as prolonged use of these products can reduce muscle tone.

Try over-the-counter medications. Anti-inflammatories like aspirin or ibuprofen can be helpful in reducing swelling that might irritate nerve roots in the spine. Consider acetaminophen to help with pain relief. Consult with your doctor to make sure it is safe for you to take these medications.

Try applying heat to the affected areas. The application of heat can help to relax your muscles. A warm bath or heating pad may also help loosen up tight muscles.
Try a sequence of alternating hot and cold packs on the affected areas. While heat works to alleviate muscle stiffness, the cold sensation may help reduce pain and discomfort. Al-

ternate between hot and cold every three minutes, repeating this pattern three times. Try doing this periodically at different times throughout your day, for a total of two or three times during the first couple days of sciatica pain.

Take steps to manage stress. Stress can have a significant impact on back pain. Breathing exercises have a calming effect and can help promote relaxation while alleviating muscle tension and rigidity. See page 12 for an example of a relaxation-promoting breathing exercise.

Stretching can help alleviate lower back pain. Consider trying some simple yoga poses, which have the added benefit of facilitating relaxation.

Complementary therapies. Acupuncture or massage can be helpful for managing pain associated with sciatica.

Stay hydrated. Be sure you're drinking enough water during the course of your day to promote healthy muscles and joints. The average is six glasses, but the most accurate test is the urine test—drink until the color of your urine is light yellow (think lemonade) to clear.

Avoid caffeine. This is especially important in the afternoon and evening, as it may contribute to dehydration and sleeplessness.

Get plenty of sleep. Although it may be difficult, especially since pain can intensify at night, do your best to give your body the rest it needs. Sleep is one of the keys to recovery. If pain is preventing you from getting a good night's rest, try changing your sleeping position. Curling up in the fetal position with a pillow between your knees, or lying on your back

Continued on next page

with a pillow under your knees, may help you rest more comfortably. Some sufferers report symptom relief by sleeping on a firmer mattress or even on the floor.

Hydrotherapy. Try immersing your body in a hot tub, jacuzzi, or even the bathtub. Hydrotherapy reduces muscle stiffness and inflammation in addition to promoting circulation. The hot water and jets, if available at home or at a local gym or spa, can help soothe nerve spasms.

Swimming. Swimming is a great way to increase blood flow to the disk and the sciatic nerve, which helps flush out the chemicals in your body causing the inflammation.

Walking. Taking short walks (between 15–20 minutes long) can stimulate blood flow and help reduce your pain.

Numbness and Weakness

Those with sciatica may feel numbness or tingling in the leg, as well as along the top of the foot and through the toes. Heaviness, tingling, and weakness can make it challenging to move one's leg or foot, and patients may experience a reduced reaction in both knee-jerk and ankle-jerk reflexes. Some people report feeling cold in the affected leg or foot.

Postural Instability

People with sciatica can experience instability in the major movement areas of the body, including the shoulders, pelvis, and ankles. A person with **postural instability** may have trouble with dynamic movements such as squatting, lunging, rotating, and bending over. Extended sitting and standing can exacerbate sciatica as well. It is important to discuss any postural instability you are experiencing with your doctor, as it can lead to an increased risk of falling and fall-related injuries, such as broken bones.

Some tips for managing postural instability include:

- Consider placing a foam roller vertically in a chair to gather feedback on your spine's position in space. Try this at work to break up extending sitting positions.
- Regularly stretch your front chest and neck muscles to promote a more upright posture.
- Try strength training exercises that focuses on the middle back and pelvis.
- Strengthen the arches of your feet. Your feet are integral in walking and balance, and controlling your upper body posture. Try this: press your heels together and position a tennis ball between the big toe mounds. Squeeze for a few seconds.

Generally, symptoms of sciatica should subside within a few days, but they may last as long as six weeks (if not longer) in some cases. If your symptoms persist, it may be an indication that you need to see a doctor.

SEEKING MEDICAL ATTENTION

If your pain continues to worsen or you develop a fever with your pain, you should contact your doctor immediately. Specific symptoms, such as increasing weakness in the leg or legs, may indicate nerve damage, so it is essential that you follow up with a healthcare professional. Similarly, if you find symptoms occur in both legs or are accompanied by bowel or bladder incontinence or dysfunction, this could be an indication of a more serious and complex condition. While 80–90 percent of patients with sciatica will get better within several weeks without the need for surgery, certain conditions may require surgical intervention, so it is important to always communicate your concerns with your doctor.

When you visit with your doctor, be sure to describe the frequency, duration, and type of pain that you are feeling. Detail for your doctor the severity of your pain and any activities (such as sitting or walking) that exacerbate it, along with any situations that relieve the pain. Note when and where the pain frequently occurs, as well as what may have caused it (such as lifting a heavy object). Your doctor should also be aware of your medical history when it comes to previous episodes of back pain and any prior injuries or accidents that involve the neck, back, or hips.

TRY IT NOW: BREATHING EXERCISES

For a simple breathing exercise, try the following. Close your eyes and take normal, deep breaths in through your nose. Concentrate on filling your lower abdomen with air. It may be helpful to place a hand on your lower abdomen to help you focus on breathing deeply and filling it. Hold that air in for 5–7 seconds, and then in a controlled, slow manner, exhale out of your mouth as silently as possible. Try this practice for approximately 5 minutes every day to help relax your body and calm your mind.

For a deep breathing exercise: Take a slow, deep breath in through your nose, and then exhale slowly through your mouth. Despite the simplicity of this breathing exercise, this technique will help slow your heart rate, relax your body, and calm your mind. So often, people grow accustomed to short, shallow breathing throughout the course of their day. Deep breathing is much more effective for the body and will lead to increased relaxation.

CHAPTER 2

Contributing Factors to Sciatic Nerve Pain

S ciatica can occur in all segments of the population, but most recent literature suggests that it is most prevalent among middle-aged individuals—defined as age 45 to 65. Nearly five million cases of sciatica are diagnosed in the United States each year, with researchers estimating that sciatic pain will affect up to 40 percent of people at some point in their lifetime.

While there are certain biological factors that predispose people to sciatica, often it is our environment and lifestyles that contribute to episodes of sciatic nerve pain. By making healthy choices with respect to diet, environment, and exercise, you can help reduce the risk of—and possibly even prevent—sciatica and other degenerative spinal conditions. Simple changes and choices that you make today can mean a big difference when it comes to back pain down the road.

WORKPLACE RISK FACTORS

The following are some common situations involving work and the workplace which can contribute to the development of sciatic pain.

Commuting

Whether taking a car, bus or train to work, commuters face a challenge every day just finding a seat that lends enough lumbar support for the average person. Most mass transportation seating is just not designed with the intention of providing comfortable support; rather, it's just meant to help you take a load off. Mass transit commuters also deal with standing in uncomfortable positions for long periods during rush hour and other busy times. While standing, their bodies are forced to stabilize against the rocking, jolting motions of the vehicle, which can be exceptionally difficult when one is trying to hold onto a pole or rail for stability.

Furthermore, trains and buses are not designed ergonomically for comfort. Often, people have to contort their bodies, whether it's getting on their tip toes or arching their backs and necks to hold onto the rails. And things only get worse when you consider that most people are usually carrying a bag of some sort. Whether it is a backpack, messenger bag or purse, these items provide additional weight that needs to be accounted for when the body tries to stabilize itself.

All these scenarios create extra compression of the discs in the spine and strain on the muscles that support it. The outcome is usually muscle spasms from lumbar asymmetry, muscular imbalances, and tight tendons that can directly irritate the sciatic nerve.

Sitting for Extended Periods

Muscular imbalances and a weak core create postural instabilities, which in turn provides a simple recipe for lower back pain and worsening sciatic pain.

Postural control refers to one's ability to maintain an upright posture and allow the body's limbs to move smoothly. This is done through the use of our core muscles, which serve as a central hub connecting our upper and lower bodies. Most motions of the body run through this central hub, either up or down; the core also serves as a power generator for these movements. A strong core not only helps generate more power, but also increases your body's ability to stabilize and balance itself. As such, a weak core places added stress on the spine and magnifies degenerative changes to the spine. This degeneration has been directly linked to worsening sciatica as the nerve is impinged upon and irritated from arthritic changes.

Sedentary lifestyles and occupations that promote prolonged sitting (such as driving) place added pressure on the discs in your back. Over time, this can weaken those discs and cause them to herniate or protrude, thereby placing additional tension on the nerves that emanate from them. Moreover, it is generally accepted by the medical community that jobs that require frequent bending, twisting and lifting of heavy loads create excess pressure on the spine and ultimately lead to instability.

(Here's a tip: Think about these factors the next time you're on vacation. Oftentimes, sciatic pain is not just from lifting a heavy bag or suitcase alone, but rather from the prolonged sitting that occurred beforehand.)

RISK FACTORS IN THE HOME

Common activities at home which can contribute to sciatic pain include:

Smoking and Excessive Alcohol Consumption

The negative health effects of tobacco smoking are far reaching and well-documented, yet many might be shocked to learn that tobacco and nicotine could play a role in their sciatic pain. Research suggests that tobacco smoking and nicotine intake reduces the molecular nutrients that keep the intervertebral discs fluid, thereby dehydrating them and making them less flexible. The consequence is a lack of protection and support for the vertebrae. These substances also limit the amount of blood flow to the discs, resulting in an impaired ability to absorb nutrients, self-repair and heal.

Similarly, excessive consumption of alcohol can have a deleterious effect in a variety of ways. Alcohol consumption is directly associated with dehydration, which can affect the discs similarly to nicotine. It also naturally slows the body's circulatory and respiratory systems, which then impairs its ability to both rid itself of toxins and replenish the nutrients needed for revitalization. Additionally, alcohol directly affects one's blood brain chemistry, which can translate to increased sensation of pain. Lastly, alcohol hinders our sleep cycles, which compromise the body's ability to repair.

The combination of these toxins culminates in a more rapid onset of degenerative disc disease and sciatic pain. Together, it provides yet one more compelling reason to quit smoking and drinking in excess, as a reduction in intake may not only delay but even prevent back pain.

Poor Posture

While having a fat wallet may be a sign of success and wealth, it may also be a harbinger of an unintended detrimental effect known as "wallet sciatica." Sitting on a wallet for prolonged periods of the day can irritate the piriformis muscle, which in turn places undue stress on the sciatic nerve (which it runs under, and sometimes through).

In addition, sitting on one elevated hip can further irritate the nerve by creating additional stress on the lumbar discs. So flatten that wallet—or better yet, carry it in your front pocket during long drives or when seated for long periods of the day.

REINFORCING THE NATURAL CURVES OF YOUR BACK

The three natural curves of your back are designed in such a way as to distribute the forces that occur naturally during activities of daily living, such as walking, running, and climbing stairs. Additionally, this functional curvature supports your head, protects the spinal cord, and acts as an anchor point for your major anatomy.

Now let's give your spine a three points of contact check-in. Sit in a chair with a straight back and position a long foam roller vertically in parallel to your spine. Position your head, middle back and pelvis in contact with the roller; these are our three points of contact. Your neck and lower back should curve forward and not contact the roller. This alignment exercise helps to remind us of healthy spinal alignment. Try this while standing as well, to help improve your standing posture.

Sleep Quality

Whether you sleep on your side, back or stomach, your sleeping position can influence sciatica. Side sleeping is the most common position, especially among women—but in this position, if the legs are too straight or drawn in too tightly, it can alter the position of the spine and exacerbate their sciatic pain. Side sleepers should therefore bend both knees slightly inwards and keep a small pillow in between their legs. This prevents the hips from twisting and placing stress on the lower back.

Sleeping on your back is often considered ideal, as it places the spine in a neutral position. In this state, the legs should stay straight so as to not place strain on the pelvis and hips. However, for those of you that sleep on your stomach, the news is not so good. This is the worst of the three positions as it places the most strain on the neck, shoulders, spine and lower back, as the spine is left unsupported.

Correcting the way you sleep may also lead you to consider the problem of your mattress selection. Choosing a mattress is a highly individualized process that can be overwhelming, leading one to feel like Goldilocks trying to figure out which mattress is just right. In general, mattresses that are too soft can cause you to sink into the bed, leaving your spine unsupported, while mattresses that are too firm may place more pressure on various trigger points in your hips and lower back. Both scenarios culminate in the same result: a poor night's sleep and pain.

UNDERSTANDING YOUR IDEAL SLEEP POSITION

According to *The Sleep Advisor* magazine, back sleepers tend to prefer a medium firm mattress, side sleepers prefer a slightly softer option, and stomach sleepers prefer a firmer mattress (to avoid sinking).

Your choice of material also makes a difference:
- Memory foams offer good contours, but can get hot. They are also great for those with partners who toss and turn, as they do not transfer energy.
- Traditional coils are durable and offer more cooling.
- Hybrids offer a combination of the first two options but are usually a lot more expensive.

It also helps to understand your body type and weight, as this will affect the firmness of the mattress you need. The heavier you are, the more support (i.e. firmness) you will need.

PHYSICAL ACTIVITY RISK FACTORS

Physical activity, or lack thereof, can increase your risk of developing sciatic nerve pain, particularly when participating in high-impact sports (such as hockey, soccer, or outdoor running).

Professional athletes and weekend warriors both—neither are immune to back pain. Those individuals participating in high impact sports such as skiing, hockey, football, soccer, gymnastics, or tennis encounter a vast array of factors that may significantly impact their sciatic pain. Whether it is from the absorption of pressure, twisting, turning or even bodily contact, the spine is placed under a great deal of stress. Not only are these actions seen on game day, but they are also repeated throughout practices in preparation for competition.

Additionally, athletes that play organized sports at all levels may ignore or trivialize their pain for fear of potential consequences. They are afraid to miss a tournament or competition, lose their position on a team or even being removed from the team; they are afraid of losing face and appearing weak in front of their teammates. It is these fears that often lead athletes to even deny symptoms, placing them at higher risk for long-term damage.

BIOLOGICAL RISK FACTORS

Finally, there are certain genetic or biological factors which play a role in determining your likelihood of sciatic issues.

Leg Length Discrepancies

Most individuals have a small difference in the length of their legs. However, those with a difference greater than 5mm are considered to be at increased risk for low back pain and worsening of their sciatic symptoms. Additionally, studies have shown that those with greater than 9mm of difference see a six fold increase in the occurrence of lower back pain episodes.

Leg length discrepancies can occur as either a functional issue or an anatomical issue. In the latter, the individual actually has one leg longer than the other, whereas the former is a result of pelvic misalignment/rotation that leads to one leg functioning as though it is longer than the other.

Foot Biomechanics

Anatomical variations in a person's feet can play an enormous role in the way they walk and how they transfer force through their joints. Researchers and podiatrists alike have long suggested a link between improper foot mechanics and lower back pain. Whether an individual pronates or supinates, has high or low arches, flat feet or even bunions, these factors change a person's biomechanical chain resulting in the impact of an everyday step leading to added stress/strain up the chain. Left uncorrected, the knees are forced to compensate to reduce the strain on the foot and ankle. In response, the hips then adjust for the knees. The result is a malrotation of the pelvis, secondary to a tightness within various tendons and muscles. While some muscles become tight and overworked, others remain weak from lack of activation.

For example, wearing high heels and unsupportive shoes can be a potential trigger. High heels tend to shift your weight

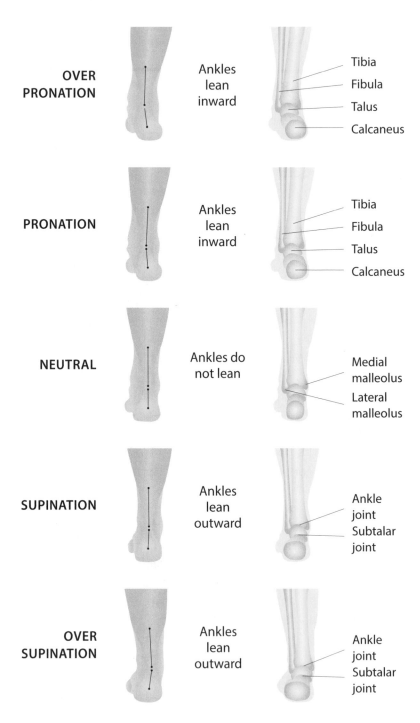

OVER PRONATION — Ankles lean inward

Tibia
Fibula
Talus
Calcaneus

PRONATION — Ankles lean inward

Tibia
Fibula
Talus
Calcaneus

NEUTRAL — Ankles do not lean

Medial malleolus
Lateral malleolus

SUPINATION — Ankles lean outward

Ankle joint
Subtalar joint

OVER SUPINATION — Ankles lean outward

Ankle joint
Subtalar joint

forward, causing you to change the natural S-curvature of your spine as your hips become flexed forward. This creates a cascade of biomechanical modifications to the body that ultimately generates tightness in the hamstrings, hip flexors and gluteal muscles. This chronically stretched position then leads to sciatic nerve irritation, given that the nerve runs along the course of the hamstrings.

Here's a tip: Check your shoes! The bottoms of your shoes may reveal an uneven wear pattern from shoe to shoe. This may be an early indication that you have an issue with your biomechanics or even a leg length discrepancy.

Being Overweight

Being overweight or obese is a known (and thankfully modifiable) risk factor for sciatica. Extra abdominal fat not only contributes to a weaker core, but it also puts excess stress on the spine, leading to arthritis and spinal stenosis. These spinal derangements can ultimately lead to sciatica.

Remember, your abdominal muscles do exist! If you are overweight and struggling with sciatic symptoms, shedding that excess belly weight may be your ticket to a pain-free existence.

Weight loss is always a sensitive issue. If you are having trouble losing weight, speak to your health care provider to develop a weight loss strategy conducive to your personal needs.

Diabetes

Uncontrolled and long-standing diabetes tend to affect the peripheral nerves of our bodies, leading to neuropathy, with patients often developing pain, numbness and tingling in their legs and feet. Although rare, there have been cases reported of diabetic sciatic neuropathy. Differentiating between the two may be difficult, and while controlling your diabetes is key, one should seek medical attention to properly discern the underlying issue.

Aging

With each year of wisdom that we accrue, we sadly also gain a year of wear and tear on our bodies. The average moderately active person takes an average of over 2.73 million steps a year. This translates to quite a bit of impact on our joints and spine. If a person is overweight or obese, that excess weight can further worsen the degenerative changes—one pound of weight correlates to approximately four pounds of pressure on our joints and spine. Furthermore, with age, the risk of arthritis increases.

Thankfully, maintaining a healthy lifestyle and body weight has been shown to limit the impact of this wear and tear. Activity is key to vitality!

Pregnancy

Pregnancy affects women in a variety of ways, some of which can contribute to the development or worsening of sciatic pain. As a woman progresses through trimesters, she inevitably gains weight and retains more fluid. This changes her center of gravity, thereby altering the shape of the lumbar spine and placing increased strain on her lower back. Additionally, hormone mediated changes cause the pelvic ligaments to relax and loosen, making it easier for the sciatic nerve to shift and be impinged upon. If this weren't enough, the growing uterus and fetus place added weight on the sciatic nerve. As the fetus descends in preparation for birth, a process that can last for weeks, the pain can become much more pervasive. Pregnancy and birth, while miraculous in nature, are a constant demonstration of the strength and fortitude of women!

MENOPAUSE AND SCIATICA

Menopause is often linked to hot flashes, mood disturbances, weight gain and difficulty sleeping. But did you know that it has also been linked to an increased risk of degenerative disk disease? Research has found that women between the ages of 50–60 have higher incidences of disc degeneration than their male counterparts. This difference may be linked to menopause's decreasing the body's production of estrogen.

Not only is estrogen essential for bone health, but it has also been shown to influence the well-being of our spinal discs. Some studies have shown that the intervertebral disc contains estrogen receptors, located on the membrane of the disc that contains and protects the cushion of the vertebrae. Decreased estrogen leads to a thinning of this surrounding membrane, reducing the ability of the vertebral disc to withstand forces of compression and torsion.

In addition, the same research suggests that estrogen also directly plays a role in the vascular supply to the disc, as estrogen opens the blood supply that feeds the disc region, allowing more nutrients rich in growth factors to reach it. A reduction in estrogen therefore indirectly results in malnutrition of the discs. Furthermore, this drop in estrogen negatively affects the bone in that it becomes weaker over time, leading to osteoporosis. The aftermath is a deterioration of the disc and bone that eventually leads to vertebral collapse and fracture.

Osteoporosis then further weakens bones by making them more porous and generally more unstable, especially in the vertebra and lumbar spine. This places individuals at greater risk for compression fractures which, along with the conditions outlined above, can pinch the sciatic nerve and cause pain.

Depression

Depression represents a constellation of symptoms that negatively influence the way a person feels, acts and thinks. It shifts the individual's reality by altering their perception of pain, self-worth and well-being. While chemical disturbances in the brain lower one's pain threshold, they also create circumstances that contribute to worsening back pain and sciatic pain.

Alterations in the brain's neurotransmitters can cause an overall lack of motivation and self-worth. Coupled with low self-esteem and a loss of energy, an environment with less physical activity and movement or prolonged sitting and laying down is created. The result is a sensation of increased fatigue and pain and tightened or weakened muscles that create more pressure on the spine and lower back.

People who suffer from depression (or even occasional bouts of depression) can develop postural anomalies, as they are more likely to sit or lay for prolonged periods, slouch, keep their shoulders rounded and hunch their necks. These problems are compounded by either sleeping too little or too much. Research has also shown that depressed patients are associated with more pain complaints and greater impairment in functional capacity. This is because pain and depression pathways act on similar neurotransmitters in the brain. Physicians will commonly use antidepressants to treat chronic pain for this reason. But while these medications have helped in many ways, they have also been implicated in unwanted weight gain, another factor that contributes to back pain.

Now that we have a more thorough understanding of the risk factors for sciatica that the average person faces in their life, at home and at work, let's take a look at some of the simple lifestyle changes you can make right now to reduce, or even eliminate, your sciatic pain.

CHAPTER 3

Improving Wellness with Lifestyle Changes

J ust as sciatica symptoms can be worsened or exacerbated by poor lifestyle choices such as bad posture and sedentary habits, symptoms can be improved and risk factors mitigated through the implementation of simple, healthy changes to your day-to-day routine. In this chapter, we'll explore some of the easiest (and most effective) ways of managing sciatica to provide relief and complement a corrective exercise program.

TIPS FOR BETTER SLEEP

As mentioned previously (see page 9), curling up in the fetal position with a pillow between your knees, or lying on your back with a pillow under your knees, may help you rest more comfortably. Some sufferers report symptom relief by sleeping on a firmer mattress and even on the floor.

Beyond your choice of mattress and sleeping position, there are a number of simple changes you can make to your nighttime routine to reduce symptoms and improve your quality of sleep.

Practice Good Sleep Hygiene
Sleep hygiene refers to the habits and activities you engage in before bed. Irregularities in routine, such as screen gazing on your phone or television, can disrupt sleep. It's best to stick to a program of nighttime habits that will signal your body that it's time to sleep. Try drinking a relaxing mug of hot tea while reading or doing a restorative meditation practice, with or without the aid of an app. Both are great ways to ease into a restful sleep.

Ice Up Before Bed
If you're having a flare up, you can always ice the sore spots before bed to help reduce pain and swelling and get a better night's sleep.

Stretch Out Before Bed
You can reduce nerve pressure by doing light stretching before bed, or even in bed. Stretches with a foam roller are particularly recommended, and can be found in the exercise section of this book.

Pick Your Spot
If you're a back sleeper, try stacking a few pillows under your knees to provide elevation, which will lessen pressure on your spine. This position "unloads" the back and hips by placing the weight of your legs on the pillows. If you're a side sleeper, bend your top knee to position it upwards, toward your head. Prop it up with two to three pillows to square off your hip position for extra relief. If you are a mover and/or a shaker, try putting a tennis ball in your pajama pocket on the side that hurts. This way, you won't roll over onto it during the night.

Mattress and Pillow Comfort

You may love a soft mattress, but your sciatica doesn't. In other words, the firmer the mattress, the better. If a new mattress isn't in your budget, try sliding a piece of plywood in between the mattress and the box spring for extra support. Or, you can try sleeping directly on the floor with a yoga mat or sheet/blanket underneath you. Don't give up after one night; it may take a few days to acclimate. You can also try using a recliner. Many patients report renting one from a local furniture store, saying it allows them to sleep through the night.

On the topic of pillow selection: it's best to keep your upper spine straight and in alignment while sleeping because pain impacts our whole body, not just one spot. That's why it's important to have good all-over support, from the neck down. Best to buy a neck support pillow rather than craning your neck with too many fluffy pillows or pillows with no support at all.

Pain Patches and Creams

If your pain is localized, try using an 8-hour pain relieving patch or rub in capsaicin or menthol cream on the sore spot before bedtime. These pain relieving gels (usually called analgesics) often contain menthol, an ingredient that blocks pain receptors and relaxes stiff muscles.

DEALING WITH SCIATICA AT WORK

Sitting

Sitting for long periods of time isn't good for your spine or your sciatica pain. If your job entails sitting all day, be sure to maintain proper posture. Use a well-designed, ergonomic swivel chair with armrests and good lower back support. You can also add low back support by placing a lumbar pillow or even a rolled-up towel at the base of your chair. It also helps to keep your feet flat on the floor (never crossed) with your knees and hips level. And, if possible, stand up every 20 minutes and walk a couple of laps around your workspace, the same as you would on an airplane.

Standing

Jobs that require workers to stand on their feet all day can also induce pain. Varying your posture is a smart way to care for your spine on the job, so mix it up whenever you can between sitting and standing. Try alternating between resting one foot and then the other on a stool or box throughout the day, changing it up every 10–15 minutes. Always try to sit at breaktime to give your spine a rest.

Sitting and Standing

Sit-to-stand desks and stand-up desks are all the rage right now—and for good reason! Studies continue to prove that the more we stand, the longer we live. Sit-to-stands enable you to adjust the height of your desk to go from sitting to standing in one easy motion, while stand-up desks allow for more variable movement. Bending at the waist to get up from your chair can stretch and aggravate an already irritable sciatic nerve. Otherwise, slide to the front of your seat and stand up by straightening your legs.

TECH TIPS FOR COMPUTER USERS

Creating a sciatica-friendly computer workstation is easier than you may think. Consider these three easy-to-incorporate tips:

1. Position the computer monitor at eye level.
2. Avoid reaching for the keyboard and mouse pad.
3. Choose a chair with excellent back support.

By incorporating each of these three things, you can avoid leaning or slumping your body forward.

Lifting

Jobs that require heavy lifting require extra care. The first rule is not to lift with your back, ever. Always engage your lower extremities using only your legs and core muscles. Keep your back straight, bend only your knees and move straight up and down without twisting. Don't be a hero by attempting to lift anything too heavy or cumbersome.

COMMUTING TIPS

We've discussed the variety of stresses your body is forced to undergo during long commutes (see page 14). There are a few easy steps you can take to mitigate these stressors, however.

Packing Ice/Heat Packs
Carrying disposable ice and/or heat packs can help you prep for any unexpected sciatica flare-ups, for example. The cold therapy can help reduce inflammation while the heat therapy stimulates heat receptors in your skin which causes your brain to focus less on your sciatic pain. Keep these packs in your carry-on luggage and in easy to reach places, such as the glove box in your car. (Be aware that disposable cold and/or heat packs are not allowed on airplanes, but you can always bring your own plastic bag and ask the flight attendant to fill it with ice.)

Lighten Your Luggage Load
Lifting and carrying heavy luggage can strain your lumbar spine (lower back) and illicit sciatica symptoms such as leg pain, or leg or foot numbness. To avoid this, you can mail your luggage ahead of time. If this is not an option, use two smaller pieces of luggage rather than one large one. If possible, replace old suitcases with wheeled luggage to minimize your need to carry suitcases over long distances.

Get Up and Move About
Believe it or not, the act of sitting puts more stress on your spine than moving about or standing.

Try moving around every 20–30 minutes by walking up and down the airplane, bus or train aisles and doing light stretching. While sitting, keep your feet on the ground and your knees at a right angle. Use cruise control while driving over long distances, and adjust your seat to different positions to keep from straining your back.

HEALTHY NUTRITION FOR SCIATICA

Next to exercise and physical activity, nutrition is the most important factor for your overall health—and for recovering from sciatica pain.

Here is a list of suggested foods to incorporate into your diet to help reduce sciatic symptoms.

Foods Rich in B Vitamins

Any foods in the vitamin B6, B12 and folate family are vital to nervous system health.

- **Vitamin B6:** Also known as pyridoxine, vitamin B6 helps metabolize your body's neurotransmitters. Foods rich in this nutrient include bananas, fish, grass fed meat, and legumes.
- **Vitamin B12:** This helps maintain healthy myelin, the fatty substance that wraps around nerve fibers to help speed up communication between neurotransmitters. Vitamin B12 can be found in pasture-raised chicken and eggs, wild-caught fatty fish such as salmon, and grass-fed dairy products.
- **Folate:** This helps produce neurotransmitters and is found in many vegetables. The best sources of folate are in asparagus, bok choy, broccoli, cauliflower, and romaine lettuce.

If you are currently taking medications, remember that foods and vitamins (even if thought to be benign and healthy) can interact with other medications in potentially harmful ways. It is always a good idea to consult with your healthcare provider before adding anything new to your daily routine.

Anti-Inflammatory Foods

There are many types of foods that may help ease your pain and swelling, which can be beneficial for sciatica. Some top choices include:

- **Spices:** Specific spices contain antioxidants that may help reduce inflammatory responses: namely cloves, ginger, rosemary, and turmeric. Try adding them to your favorite dishes and see if you experience relief.
- **Dark leafy greens:** Vegetables such as collard greens, kale, spinach, and Swiss chard contain antioxidants that can help fight cellular damage.
- **Green tea:** Japanese matcha tea contains 17 times more antioxidants than wild blueberries, which are also rich in antioxidants.
- **Fermented vegetables:** Foods such as kimchi, miso, natto, pickles, and sauerkraut are good for gut health which helps boost your immune system and ward off internal inflammation. Fermented dairy products such as kefir and yogurt are also good options.

Muscle-Repair Foods

Muscle problems can cause sciatica, as in the case of a tight piriformis muscle. Certain foods work to help repair and nourish your muscles to help prevent future injuries, such as:

- **Nuts and seeds:** These little gems contain plant-based omega-3 fatty acids to help guard against and fight inflammation, in addition to adding protein for muscle synthesis and growth.
- **Pasture-raised eggs:** Eggs contain generous amounts of protein to help repair and strengthen your muscles, as well as enhance energy production.
- **Tart cherries:** This small fruit packs a powerful punch in helping to decrease muscle pain and inflammation.
- **Wild-caught salmon:** The omega-3s found in this fish group contain lean protein for building and strengthening muscles.

Note: Be sure to eat proteins in moderation (1 gram for every kilogram of your lean body mass) to lower the risk of stimulating your mTOR (mammalian target of rapamycin), a marker linked to cancer from the overconsumption of protein.

SCIATICA SELF-CARE

In addition to increased exercise, improved nutrition and simple lifestyle changes, a bit of healthy self-care can go a long way in easing and reducing sciatica symptoms. Although resting for a day or so may provide some relief, prolonged inactivity will make your signs and symptoms worse, so whenever possible, try some of the following options instead:

Cryotherapy treatments. The benefits of cold packs on sciatic pain has been discussed previously, but there's also the option of whole body cryotherapy. Cryotherapy has received quite a bit of endorsement from celebrities and athletes, and involves the use of freezing or near freezing temperatures which preliminary studies suggest can reduce inflammation, promote healing and temporarily reduce pain. While these benefits need to be further substantiated, cryotherapy presents another non-invasive measure that one can employ in the fight against sciatic pain. (If you have high blood pressure, heart or lung disease, troubles with poor circulation, neuropathy or allergies triggered by the cold, you should consult with a physician before utilizing this approach.)

Stretching. Practicing stretching exercises for your lower back can help you feel better and might help relieve nerve root compression. Avoid jerking, bouncing or twisting during the stretch, and try to hold the stretch for at least 30 seconds.

TENS units. Transcutaneous electrical nerve stimulation (TENS) units are another non-invasive and portable option for pain relief. These hand-held devices deliver small electrical impulses conducted through electrodes with adhesive pads that are attached to a person's skin. These impulses inundate the nervous system with electrical signals, decreasing its ability to transmit pain signals to the spinal cord and brain. Additionally, it helps the body to produce endorphins, its own natural pain reliever. While these machines are purported to reduce muscle spasms and provide pain relief for up to 24 hours, studies have provided conflicting results. Before utilizing these machines, you should consult with a physician as to whether it is medically appropriate.

Over-the-counter medications. Pain relievers such as ibuprofen (Advil, Motrin IB, others) and naproxen sodium (Aleve) are sometimes helpful for sciatica.

MEDICAL TREATMENT OPTIONS

If your pain doesn't improve with self-care measures, your doctor might suggest some of the following treatments:

Medications
Common symptoms of sciatica may respond well to certain types of medication, in concert with the above lifestyle changes. The types of drugs that might be prescribed for sciatica pain include:

- Anti-inflammatories
- Muscle relaxants
- Narcotics
- Tricyclic antidepressants
- Anti-seizure medications

Remember, long term use of these medications can have detrimental effects on your stomach and even blood pressure. Please consult with your physician if you are utilizing these medications on a regular basis.

Physical Therapy
Once your acute pain improves, your doctor or a physical therapist can design a rehabilitation program to help you prevent

future injuries. This typically includes exercises to correct your posture, strengthen the muscles supporting your back, and improve your flexibility. The goal of physical therapy is to achieve a certain level of function that minimizes pain, enhances quality of life, and teaches the patient strategies to incorporate into their daily lives. Physical therapy is generally covered through health insurance, so there may be limitations on the amount and frequency of sessions available to you.

Steroid Injections

In some cases, your doctor might recommend an injection of a corticosteroid medication into the area around the involved nerve root. Corticosteroids help reduce pain by suppressing inflammation around the irritated nerve. The effects usually wear off in a few months. The number of steroid injections you can receive is limited, however, as the risk of serious side effects increases when the injections occur too frequently.

Surgery

This option is usually reserved for when the compressed nerve causes significant weakness, loss of bowel or bladder control, or when you have pain that progressively worsens or doesn't improve with other therapies. Surgeons can remove the bone spur or the portion of the herniated disk that is pressing on the pinched nerve.

Alternative Medicine

In addition to traditional medical practices, alternative therapies commonly used for low back pain include:

Acupuncture. In acupuncture, the practitioner inserts hair-thin needles into your skin at specific points on your body. Some studies have suggested that acupuncture can help back pain, while others have found no benefit. If you decide to try acupuncture, choose a licensed practitioner to ensure that he or she has had extensive training.

Chiropractic. Spinal adjustment (manipulation) is one form of therapy chiropractors use to treat restricted spinal mobility. The goal is to restore spinal movement and, as a result, improve function and decrease pain. Spinal manipulation appears to be as effective and safe as standard treatments for low back pain, but might not be appropriate for radiating pain. Additionally, chiropractors may employ deep tissue techniques designed to loosen tight muscles, thereby relieving muscle spasms contributing to sciatic pain.

Yoga

Yoga is a movement-based activity that involves static and dynamic poses, and which can provide some benefit to sciatica sufferers. All major movement areas are utilized during yoga, including the shoulder girdle, hip girdle, and ankle joints. (These major anatomy points connect to bony landmarks located in proximity to these areas of movement.)

The shoulder girdle, to give an example, is used during many yoga movements that involve stability, such as upward/downward dog, planks, and push-ups. The shoulders are especially relevant to sciatica because instability in this area may cause increased movement in the lower back and hip girdle to compensate. Focusing on developing strength in the chest, shoulders, and ribcage allow the core and hips to remain stable, and avoids placing undo strain on the pelvis.

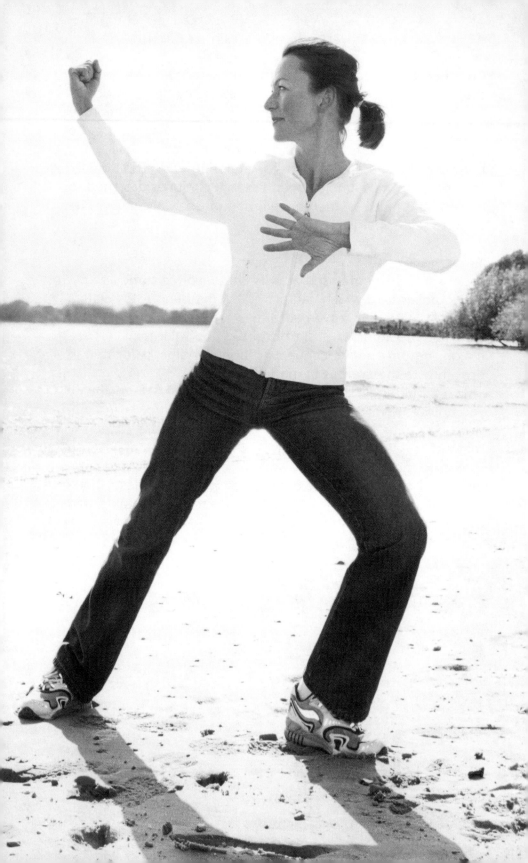

CHAPTER 4

Improving Wellness with Exercise

Regular physical activity is essential to maintaining overall health and wellness in all stages of life, and keeping to a regular exercise program can help manage, delay, or even prevent a variety of health problems. The numerous benefits of exercise are well-documented: regular physical activity can boost your mood, strengthen your muscles and bones, and help improve flexibility and mobility. For these reasons, it is especially important for someone with sciatica to regularly engage in exercise and physical activity.

Sciatica is a condition that responds extremely well to healthy movement strategies, particularly when done as a daily habit. Research has found that regular exercise—using the proper form—may be an effective strategy to lessen the frequency and severity of sciatica. In some cases, exercise can even prevent sciatica from occurring at all. In addition, when patients engage in a regular program of gentle exercises, they can often recover more quickly from sciatica pain and are less likely to have flare ups.

Note that in some cases, individuals struggling with the back and leg pain associated with sciatica may not feel inclined to engage in vigorous exercise. In cases like these, it is beneficial to work with your doctor or physical therapist in conjunction with an exercise specialist to find a workout program that is suited to your individual needs and goals. If you experience recurrent or chronic back pain (generally defined as pain that lasts for over 90 days), we recommend having a consultation with your primary care provider and/or physical therapist, who can better advise you on appropriate exercises for your condition. They may recommend physical therapy over an independent workout regimen, which incorporates a combination of strengthening, stretching, and aerobic conditioning.

HOW DOES EXERCISE BENEFIT PEOPLE LIVING WITH SCIATICA?

All people with sciatica, regardless of how frequent or severe their episodes of back pain are, should consider beginning a workout routine. And the earlier, the better: people often wait until they have mobility problems or back pain to begin exercising, but the sooner a person begins an exercise program designed to reduce sciatic pain and prevent or delay the onset of future episodes of sciatica, the more effective the program will be. Exercise can help improve mobility and strengthen the areas involved, so that people with sciatica can either eliminate future episodes altogether or at least lower the intensity and frequency of any future episodes.

Other ways exercise can benefit people with sciatica include:

- Improved flexibility
- Building healthy, strong bones
- Increased awareness of proper body alignment and mechanics

- Increased strength, especially in core stabilizing muscles like the back, which support the spine and remove pressure from the spinal discs
- Improved circulation to better distribute nutrients through the body, including to the spinal discs
- Releases endorphins which can naturally alleviate pain
- Reduced fatigue and increases energy levels
- A greater sense of well-being and improved self-esteem
- Improved ability to perform tasks
- Controls weight and burns calories
- Improved sleep quality

WHAT TYPES OF EXERCISES BEST HELP WITH SCIATICA?

The exercises outlined in Chapter 5 have been carefully selected to improve mobility, increase flexibility, and strengthen muscles. These exercises target a range of symptoms, including but not limited to:

- Hip pain
- Lower back pain
- Gluteal pain
- Weakness or numbness

Keep in mind that as you begin any new exercise program, it is important to start slowly and pace yourself. As you get more comfortable over time, you can begin to increase the intensity of your workouts. Always pay attention to how your body is responding to an exercise routine and only increase frequency and intensity when your body is ready for it. Pay attention to your symptoms and take breaks if you need to do so, but above all do not give up. You have so much to gain from a well-planned exercise program, including increased energy, improved balance and mobility, and a better quality of life.

Sciatica exercises usually focus on three key areas: strengthening, stretching, and aerobic conditioning. These types of exercise may be done separately or in combination; examples of exercise that may include both strengthening and stretching include yoga, tai chi, and Pilates. And for anyone in chronic pain or with a relatively high level of sciatica pain, a good option for gentle exercise is water therapy, which is a controlled, progressive exercise program done in a warm pool.

Strengthening Exercises

There are many exercises which can help strengthen the spinal column and the supporting muscles, ligaments, and tendons. Most of these back-centric exercises focus not only on the lower back, but also the abdominal (stomach) muscles and gluteus (buttock) and hip muscles.

In addition to the back, building up strong core muscles can provide pain relief for sciatica sufferers by helping to support the spine, keeping it in alignment and facilitating movements that extend or twist the spine with less chance of injury or damage.

Stretching Exercises

Stretching is usually recommended to alleviate sciatic pain. Stretches for sciatica are designed to target those muscles that cause pain when they are tight and inflexible. For example, hamstring stretching is almost always an important part of a sciatica exercise program. Most people do not stretch these muscles (which extend from the pelvis to the knee in the back of the thigh) in their daily activities. Another stretch that is often helpful in easing sciatica is the Bird Dog, in which individuals get down on their hands and knees and extend one arm and the opposite leg, alternating between them.

When incorporating stretching exercises for the treatment of sciatic symptoms, another helpful technique is nerve flossing. Also called nerve gliding, these are gentle stretching exercises intended to stretch irritated nerves to reduce pain and improve range of motion. Gently flexing and extending one of your legs, while keeping your other muscles relaxed, is one example of nerve flossing.

Low-Impact Aerobic Exercise
Including some form of low-impact cardiovascular exercise, such as walking, swimming, or pool therapy, is common as a component of sciatic recovery. Aerobic activity encourages the exchange of fluids and nutrients in the body to help create a better healing environment, and also has the unique benefit of releasing endorphins, the body's natural pain killers, which helps reduce sciatic pain.

To Improve Strengthening
Push-ups, pg. 96
Deadbug, pg. 100
Supermans, pg. 116

To Increase Flexibility
Scissor Stretch, pg. 68
Thoracic Flex, pg. 61
Knee to Forehead (Single Knee or Double), pg. 63

To Improve Posture
Alphabet Series, pgs. 85-87
Cranial Release, pg. 62
Lateral Plank, pg. 95

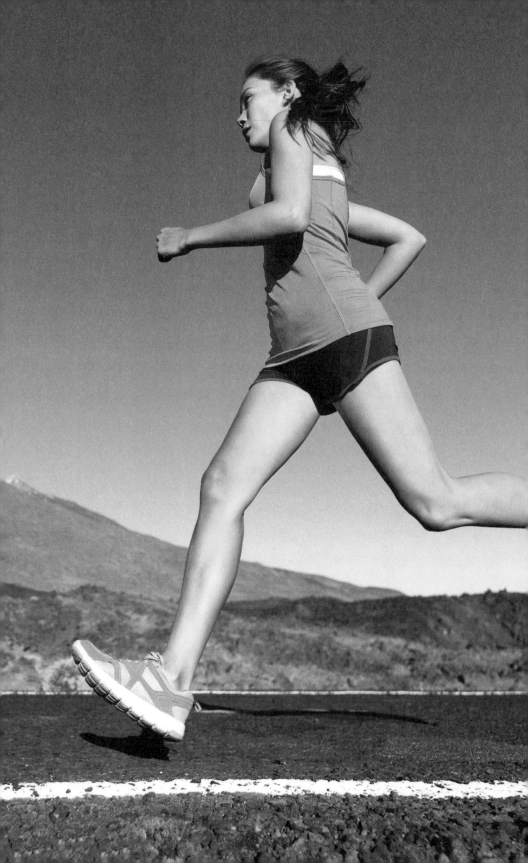

CHAPTER 5

Rules of the Road: Exercise Precautions

I n the following chapter, you will find a series of exercises carefully selected to help people with sciatica reduce pain and limit future episodes. These exercises target improved mobility, increased flexibility, and strength training. The exercises and accompanying programs are designed to be safe and effective for people with back pain. Remember: the best exercises are the ones that can be performed consistently over a number of years. In order to experience the benefits of physical activity, you must commit to regular exercise over an extended period of time.

In performing these exercises, you will be participating in a process called motor learning. This process is broken down into several stages, or phases, as you come to better understand the exercise and your body's ability to complete the movement. The first few weeks of the program are called the **cognitive** (or verbal) stage, during which you will be developing a general understanding of what to do and how to do it. This stage generally lasts 3–4 weeks. During the second stage, the **associative** stage, you will be able to perform the movements, but there may be some errors or flaws in your form. This stage usually lasts anywhere from 2–3 weeks. The final stage, the **autonomous** stage, is when you are able to perform the exercises with proper technique and can repeat sets and reps week after week without error or issue.

It is important to remember that whenever you try something new, frustration is a natural part of the process. This is particularly important as stress and frustration can exacerbate the symptoms of sciatica, so you must be patient as you learn new physical and mental exercises.

FEAR AND EXERCISE: ADDRESSING THE MIND-BODY CONNECTION

Stress, anxiety and fear cause our bodies to react in a variety of ways. This is natural: our thoughts, feelings and actions illicit responses from our bodies, which can be positive or negative. But this relationship between the mind and body is incredibly important when it comes to exercise, as it means that our minds can essentially affect how healthy we feel.

This connection is especially present when it comes to pain, as powerful memories associated with pain can create behaviors of avoidance. According to the fear avoidance model of chronic pain, "During a musculoskeletal pain episode, anxiety, pain-related fear, and pain catastrophizing interact to determine whether an individual will resume normal activities (low psychological distress) or will avoid normal activities due to anticipation of increased pain and/or re-injury (high psychological distress)." The higher the psychological distress, the worse the clinical outcomes, and the more likely the individual is to experience depressive symptoms, increased pain intensity, greater physical impairments and continued disability.

This leads to a behavior known as pain catastrophizing, in which an individual becomes fixated on their pain (i.e., not being able to stop thinking about how bad the pain is), magnifies their pain (i.e., becomes afraid that something more serious will occur) and feels helpless to manage their pain (i.e., nothing can make the pain stop). This concept affects how individuals experience pain and can often leave a person feeling paralyzed. It is this construct that leads to behavior avoidance.

The same occurs when starting an exercise program, particularly one intended to help strengthen or rehabilitate someone suffering from a painful disorder like sciatica. After experiencing pain during a workout or exercise, you develop a strong aversion to trying it again, and become unwilling to continue. Understanding why your pain is present, what worsens it, and any physical limitations it may cause is essential to confronting the fear. Individuals who confront their pain experience and progressively resume physical activities, testing and correcting their pain expectations, subsequently experience recovery in their pain symptoms.

Dealing with pain is not easy, but by incorporating some self-help techniques, you can improve. Start by:

1. Always remembering that you are in control of the pain and not the other way around.

2. Using visual imagery to see yourself pain-free, feeling well and at ease. Keep this image in your mind and let all the positive emotions associated with this image encompass you.

3. Using mindfulness techniques to "dull the pain" by focusing on controlling your fear and anxiety. Mindfulness has been long documented to have positive benefits on pain and mood. Diaphragmatic breathing, meditation, yoga and tai-chi are all common examples.

Continued on next page

4. Using positive affirmations when you feel the first inclinations of fear or pain. Repeat these positive sayings ("I can do this", "I am tougher than the pain") to yourself over and over as you focus on slowing your breathing and heart rate. This positivity, coupled with mindfulness techniques, will allow you to push past the fear.

5. Believing that you can move your body, even if there is some pain. Believe that this will make it stronger and that you will ultimately experience less pain once your body has regained its natural strength. Try to progressively get back to doing the activities you enjoy and with the people you enjoy them with. These things will help increase your confidence in yourself.

6. Understanding that you are not alone and that your clinical team (physician, therapists, trainers, etc.) are all there to help you with this pain.

EXERCISE ESSENTIALS CHECKLIST

In addition to having the proper mindset to begin a new exercise routine, it's equally important to be sure your space and equipment are also prepped and ready to go. It helps to run down a simple checklist, to make sure everything is in order.

Exercise Preparation
Exercise location: Is your environment safe, clean, and free from debris?

Proper footwear: Are you wearing proper athletic footwear (see below)?

Comfortable athletic wear: Do you have clothes that allow for freedom of movement?

Hydration: Be sure to drink six glasses of water during the course of your day.

Exercise Equipment

Rolled-up towel: Can be used for resistance training, balancing on the floor, etc.

Mirror: Provides visual feedback on cueing and technique

Dumbbells: 5–10-pound range is generally appropriate

TheraBand: Light-colored bands offer less resistance and dark-colored bands offer more resistance.

Physioball: Inflate the ball to the point where you can press your thumb on the surface without it sinking in.

Tennis ball or racquetball: For hand and foot therapy.

Foam roller: A half roller and full-length roller to release muscle tightness and treat trigger points.

USING PROPER FOOTWEAR

Your feet are an often-overlooked area of the body. Your big toe, arch, and heel are the three primary areas involved in foot strikes, balance, walking, and running, and depending on the design of your foot—whether it's flat, neutral, or high arch—you'll need different support.

Lay a towel on the bathroom floor and, when stepping out of the shower, look to see the shape of your foot on the towel. A flat foot will leave a full foot mark, whereas a small mark is indicative of a high arch. Use this information and validate it with proper footwear at a running store (or, if access is available, see a podiatrist). Wearing the proper footwear, which protects and supports your specific type of foot, will help you avoid unnecessary injury or stress during workouts.

IMPORTANT SAFETY PRECAUTIONS

In this section, you will find practical safety precautions to ob-serve when exercising. Take the time to read them carefully and incorporate them into your routine. Please be advised that it is essential you see your healthcare provider regularly for check-ups, especially before beginning any new fitness regimen.

Body positioning. Brace your core, achieve proper alignment, feel the placement of your feet, and always move from your core first before moving your limbs.

Keep a health journal. Record how you are feeling on any given day, along with the activities you did during that time. You should also record what kinds of exercises you did on each day, and how you felt both during and after your exercise session. Keeping track of this information will help you better under-stand your own health and track your progress.

Rate of Perceived Exertion (RPE). You can use the chart below to gauge how hard you are working during your session. The corresponding numerical values may also be helpful for you to record in your health journal, should you choose to keep one. These values are included in the workout programs as an in-dicator of how much effort you should be expending in each routine.

1	No Exertion at All
2	Extremely Light
3	Very Light
4	Moderate Light
5	Light
6	Moderate Hard
7	Hard (Heavy)
8	Very Hard
9	Extremely Hard
10	Full Exertion

Talk Test. This is another useful way to determine how hard you are working. As you exercise, gauge how easily you are able to converse. If you can carry a conversation with ease while exercising, you are likely working aerobically, which means your body is using oxygen as its primary energy source. If you can work aerobically for 30–45 minutes, your body will begin using fat as an energy source, which is an excellent foundation for building your exercise program.

Anaerobic work, characterized as medium intensity, should be introduced eight weeks into your exercise program. Examples include hill walking, bike sprints, etc. When performing anaerobic exercise, you may notice your leg muscles starting to feel a bit tight; your chest will expand, you will begin to sweat, and your heart rate will reach about 40–50 beats above your resting heart rate.

DETERMINING YOUR HEART RATE

To determine your heart rate, place the tips of your index, second and third fingers on your wrist, below the base of your thumb. You can also place the tips of your index and second fingers on your neck, along either side of your windpipe. During exercise, it is recommended that you find your pulse on your wrist, rather than on your neck.

When pressing lightly with your fingers, you should be able to feel your pulse. If you don't feel your pulse, move your fingers around slightly until you find it. Count the number of beats you feel in 10 seconds. Using that number, calculate your heart rate with the formula below:

(Beats in 10 seconds) x 6 = (Heart rate)

Adults over 18 years of age typically have a resting heart rate of 60–100 beats per minute. To better understand your own heart rate, you should check your pulse both before and immediately after exercising. This will give you a better idea of what your body normally does at rest, and what level your heart should be working at during an exercise session.

Calculating Your Target Heart Rate

Your target heart rate is the level of exertion you should aim for when exercising in order to gain the most benefits from your workout. Your target heart rate is also a useful range for how your body is responding to exercise. Your target heart rate is 60–80 percent of your maximum heart rate, depending on what level of exertion you wish to work at.

DIFFERENT TRAINING ZONES

Below is a list of the different levels of exertion and the corresponding percentage you would reference to determine your target heart rate. Please note, heart rate can be influenced by many different factors including sleep, stimulants, and stress. Keeping a record of your heart every few weeks combined with your RPE is a more well-rounded benchmark.

Recovery Zone (60–70 percent). Recovery training should fall into this zone (ideally at the lower end). It is also useful for very early pre-season and closed season cross-training when the body needs to recover and replenish.

Aerobic Zone (70–80 percent). Exercising in this zone will help develop your aerobic system and, in particular, your ability to transport and utilize oxygen. Continuous or rhythmic endurance training, like running and hiking, should fall in this heart rate zone.

Anaerobic Zone (80–90 percent). Training in this zone will help to improve your body's ability to deal with lactic acid. It may also help to increase your lactate threshold.

You can use the formulas below to calculate your maximum heart rate and then to find your target heart rate.

220 – age = Maximum heart rate

(Maximum heart rate) x (training percentage) = Target heart rate

For example, if a 50-year-old woman wishes to train at 70 percent of her maximum heart rate, she would use the below calculations:

$$220 - 50 = 170$$
$$170 \times 70\% = 119$$

She would thus aim to reach a heart rate of 119 during her exercise in order to work at her target heart rate.

THE KARVONEN FORMULA

We can also use the Karvonen Formula to determine target heart rate. The Karvonen Formula, named for Finnish scientist Dr. M.J. Karvonen, is based on both your maximum heart rate and resting heart rate.

Here's an example:

$$220 - 40 = 180$$
$$180 - 60 = 120$$
$$120 \times .60 \text{ (\% training range)} = 72$$
$$72 + 60 = 132$$

220 = Maximum Heart Rate
40 = Age
60 = Resting Heart Rate
.60 or 60% = Percentage Range
72 = Heart Rate Reserve
72 + 60 = Low end of heart rate training zone

The Karvonen formula is a more personalized approach, as it takes into account both age and resting heart rate.

ASSESSMENT AND SCREENING

Before beginning any exercise program, it's important to establish a baseline. This baseline provides you with a foundation to interpret ongoing feedback on your progress. Thankfully, the world of human movement science includes a seemingly endless variety of screenings, tests and evaluations that can provide useful data, tailored to a specific audience.

In the case of sciatica, the patient using this program is understood to have gone through an evaluation with their primary care provider (during your annual physical or, if symptomatic, on an episodic basis) to discuss ongoing symptoms such as referral pains, localized back pain, or difficulty sitting for extended periods of time.

If you are struggling with ongoing pain, your primary care provider may suggest seeing a physiatrist, a physician specializing in rehabilitation medicine. The results of their evaluation may determine whether you are cleared for physical activity and, if so, what next steps are recommended (including working with a community-based provider such as a physical therapist or personal trainer).

Activities of Daily Living

The deciding factor in a care provider or physiatrist evaluation will often be level of pain and/or difficulties with the activities of daily living (ADLs). We recognize that some of our readers may have limitations related to sciatica that make activities of daily living more challenging; for these individuals, it is all the more important to establish benchmarks to measure improvement. (Remember, however, that improvement is relative so don't get discouraged if you're not measuring up to someone else's standard—everyone can make strides by establishing a daily regimen.)

Basic Activities of Daily Living (ADLs). Basic ADLs are those tasks we perform on a daily basis. These tasks are generally self-care related in nature, and include things like bathing, dressing and feeding oneself, personal hygiene, and toilet hygiene.

Instrumental Activities of Daily Living (IADLs). Instrumental ADLs involve slightly more complex uses of the body's functional mobility, and typically feature multiple basic ADLs being performed simultaneously. IADLs are relevant to sciatica treatment in that sciatic pain affects muscle control, rigidity, and ultimately compensatory posture (i.e. a forward lean) as a result of an altered gait pattern (think shuffling as compared to normal strides).

Postural conditions can impact one's ability to perform these activities; for example, the inability to raise one's arm above their head due to rounded shoulders or kyphosis prohibiting one from being able to place dishes in a cabinet. Likewise, a limited ability to bend over (using proper squat mechanics) without low back pain makes it much more difficult to pick something up off of the floor.

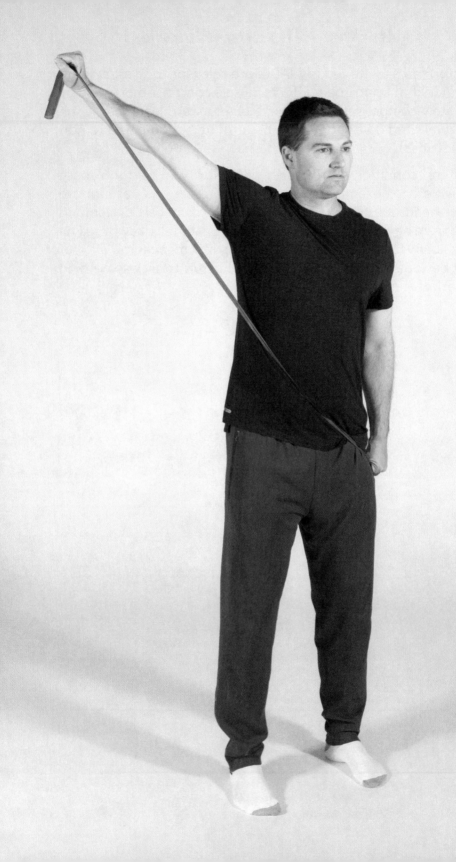

CHAPTER 6

The Exercises

In selecting the perfect exercises to aid in both general and targeted sciatica improvement, adopting a comprehensive movement approach is paramount. The exercises featured in this book take into account the fact that sciatica is a condition where maintaining movement quality can be difficult during periods of acute sciatic pain.

These exercises were purposely selected with an eye towards balancing all three planes of movement: frontal (side to side), sagittal (front to back), and transverse (rotational). By working these planes individually or in combination, we allow for a never-ending selection of program possibilities, as well as countless exercises to choose from.

The concept of exercise relies on structure, and for good reason: there are specific techniques and forms necessary to perform each movement correctly. That being said, there is also a fun, unstructured aspect to daily movement that allows us to express ourselves in ways a machine, dumbbell, or TheraBand could never accomplish.

BENCHMARKS

Our benchmarks are practical. We establish three categories of assessment that cast a wide net, related to sciatica.

Our assessment categories are as follows:

Mobility. Mobility is a general term covering flexibility, balance, and general body control. As we age, it's generally thought that our movement quality decreases due to loss of muscle strength, toning and slowing of reflexive response. Fortunately, through healthy living movement quality can be relatively maintained.

Physical. Physical benchmarking means establishing clear markers for strength and endurance. Improvements in this category trickle over into the mobility and activities of daily living assessments. Building strength tends to produce positive changes in body composition, toning, and reflexes.

Activities of Daily Living (ADLs). ADLs are activities we perform every day, regardless of age, gender, physical status, or occupation. Your sciatica recovery program is only as effective as the degree to which it supports positive lifestyle changes related to your condition.

STABILITY VS. MOBILITY

A few things to bear in mind, given the importance we'll be placing on mobility and range of movement in this program. The body's movements consist of alternating patterns of "stability and mobility." By design, joints have primary actions such as hinging, rotation, and flexion. Corresponding to the action is their innate action for stability or mobility.

Below are some examples, as well as the category they traditionally fall under:

- **Feet:** Stability. Feet support the load of the body.
- **Ankles:** Mobility. Ankles move forward and backward to propel the body.
- **Knees:** Stability. Knees act as a stable connector to the major bones above and below. They assist in supporting the load of the body by their location in the lower extremity.
- **Hips:** Mobility.
- **Lower Spine:** Stability.

THE EXERCISES

The following section presents each exercise featured in this book's program. The description for each exercise looks to provide a detailed understanding of how to perform the given exercise. Each exercise also includes a "Feel It Here" note, indicating where in your body you should most feel the effects of the movement.

Gastroc Roller

FEEL IT HERE: Lower Legs

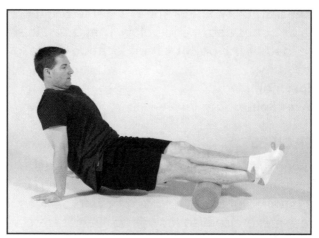

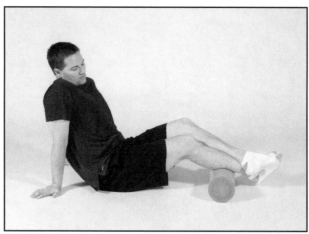

Begin the movement sitting on the floor. Extend your legs in front of you, about hip-width apart. Place the back of your lower leg on the roller and locate a spot that is slightly uncomfortable between the ankle and back of the knee. Hold, rotating the ankle to increase pressure, before moving on to the next spot. To increase pressure, stack the opposite leg on top.

Quad Roller

FEEL IT HERE: **Upper Legs**

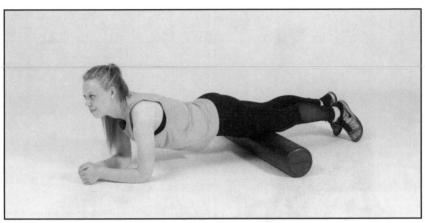

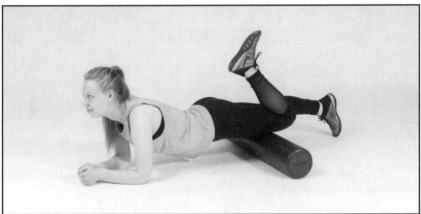

Start by positioning the foam roller on the front of the thighs. Keep your core braced. Flex and extend one knee at a time, moving to the next point on the thigh.

Glute Roller

FEEL IT HERE: Glutes

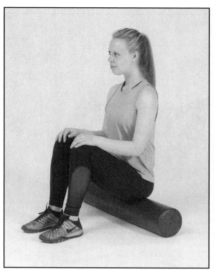 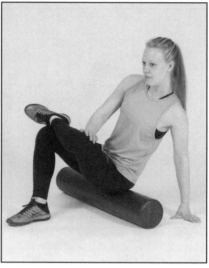

Begin by sitting on the roller. Shift your body weight to one hip while crossing over the same side ankle. Gently begin making small circles with the hip on the roller. Use your knee to assist in deepening the release.

Thoracic Flex

FEEL IT HERE: Mid-section

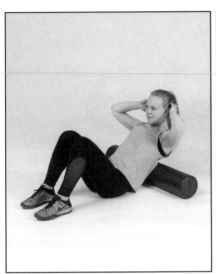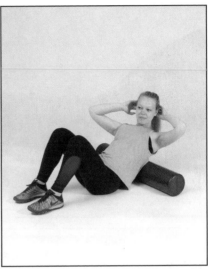

You can use a full roller, half roller, or thick, rolled up towel. Position the roller immediately below your shoulder blades. Your elbows should be pointed to the sides. Feel the foam roller pressing against your middle spine. Keep your ribs heavy into the ground so the core muscles are active and working through the entire motion. Your front abs will be working the entire time but the latter muscles, namely the obliques, are the actual movers.

Cranial Release

FEEL IT HERE: Neck, Head

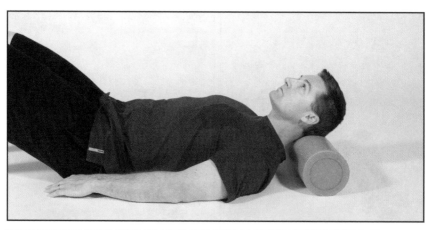

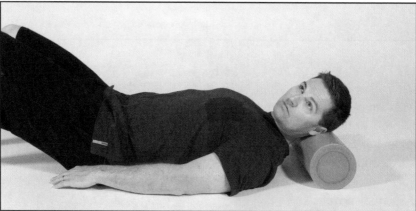

Lay on your back. Position the back of your head, right where it meets the base of your neck, on the roller. You should be in a comfortable position; draw your feet into your hips if needed. Your hands should be relaxed near the sides of your hips. If you need to stabilize the roller, place your hands on the sides of the roller. Rotate your head to the right and left. When rotating your head to the right and left, feel the small space that sits on either side of your head. Keep pressure in the roller by slightly extending your neck, emphasizing proper alignment.

Knee to Forehead
(Single Knee or Double)

FEEL IT HERE: Hips

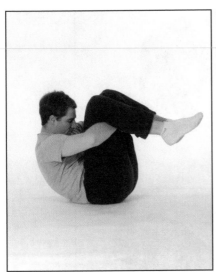 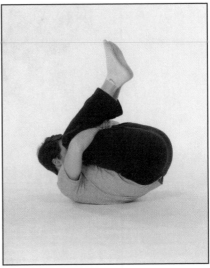

Tighten up your stomach. Draw the knee towards the chest, grabbing the knee with two hands.

Prayer Pose

FEEL IT HERE: Shoulders, Back

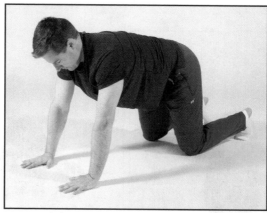

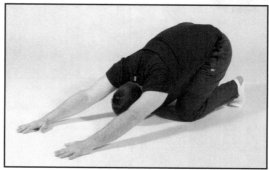

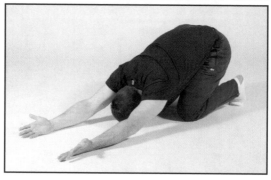

Begin in a kneeling position and reach through under the opposite side.

Straight Leg Hamstring Stretch
FEEL IT HERE: Back of Legs, Lower Back

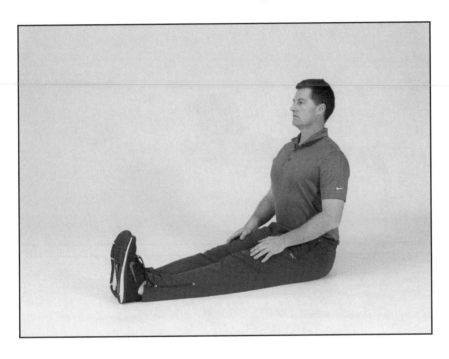

Sitting upright with your legs in front, tilt your hips forward like a water bucket, making sure you are not experiencing any discomfort or pain. As you tilt forward, feel the stretch behind your legs. If you have difficulty sitting upright, rest your back against a wall.

Ribcage Opener
FEEL IT HERE: Shoulders, Mid-section

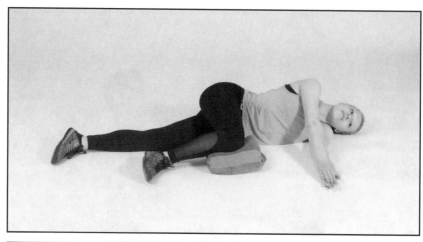

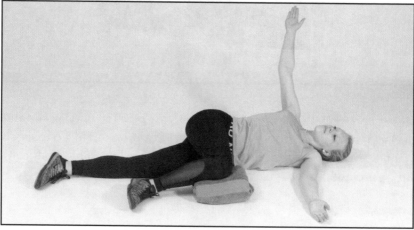

Lay on the ground and position a rolled-up towel or foam roller under your knee. Start with your hands together. Press your knees into the object then initiate rotation with your hand. Follow the rotation down the arm until you feel it through your ribcage.

Ribs Heavy

FEEL IT HERE: Mid-section

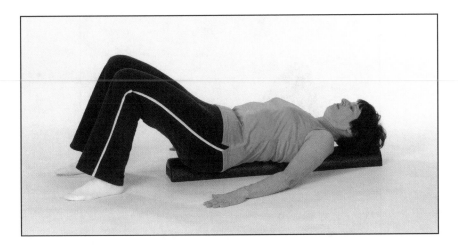

Use a foam roller or towel rolled up lengthwise. Make sure your head, middle back, and hips are in contact with the roller or towel. Feel your lower ribs make contact with the roller, yet make sure you have space in your lower back. This movement replaces pushing your lower back into the ground or flattening out your lower back during core movements, and will be applied to all exercises. When lying on your back, the body should contact the floor at your head, shoulders, hips, upper legs and calves. Your neck, lower back, and space behind your knees should be off the floor.

Scissor Stretch

FEEL IT HERE: Legs, Hips

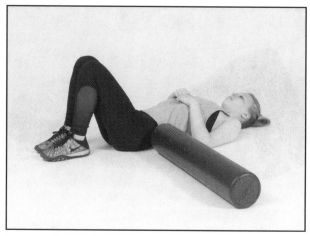

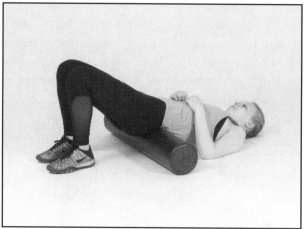

Lay on your back with your knees bent and feet close to your hips. Press your feet into the floor, then elevate your hips. Slide a foam roller (or very thick towel) beneath your tailbone/sacrum.

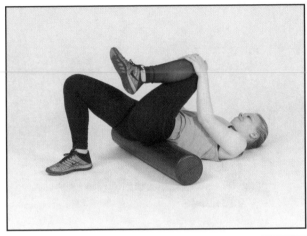

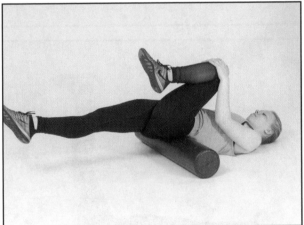

Keeping your ribs heavy, pull one knee to your chest and hold. Extend the leg next, keeping ribs heavy, engaging the core. The sacrum is the flattish bone that positions itself directly below the lower back. Place the palm of your hand on the sacrum; it should fit nicely.

Single Leg Hamstring Stretch
FEEL IT HERE: Legs, Hips

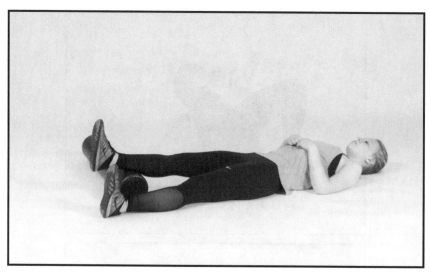

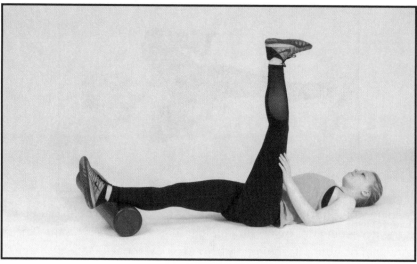

Begin by lying on your back, with a foam roller positioned beneath your hamstring. Straighten out the leg being stretched, while pressing the non-stretching leg into the ground.

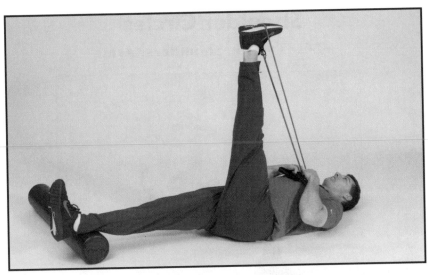

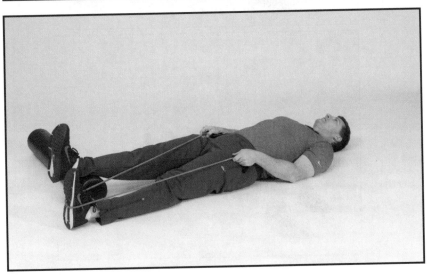

Modifications for this exercise include the use of a band. Lie on the floor with your legs extended in front of you. Loop an elastic band around the ball of one foot and raise your leg by pulling the band toward you while keeping your knee straight.

Shoulder Circles

FEEL IT HERE: Shoulders, Arms

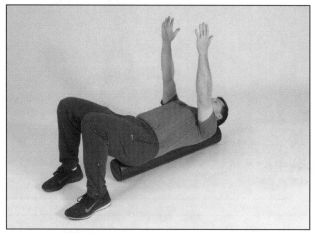

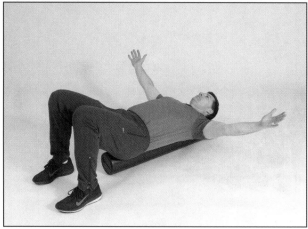

Lay down on the roller with your spine resting in the long position. If you need increased balance during the movement use a half roller or rolled up towel. Feel pressure on your spine. Only your head, middle back, and pelvis should be resting in contact with the roller. Initiate smooth circles with your arms as if you have a dinner tray in each hand.

Squat with Reach Across

FEEL IT HERE: Hips, Core

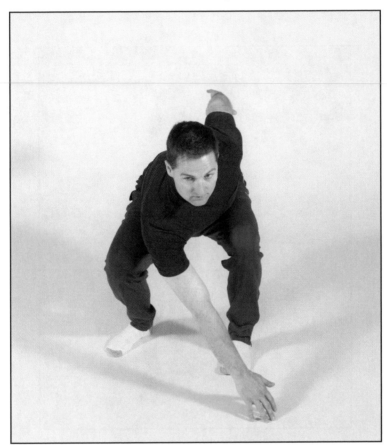

Begin by standing in a neutral stance. Squat down by dropping your hips back as if sitting in a chair. Reach across your body in front of the opposite side foot. This reach across will enhance activation of the hip muscle, decreasing the strain on the knee.

Calf Raise/Shin Raise
FEEL IT HERE: Calves, Legs

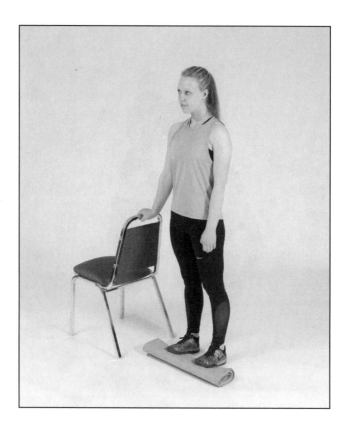

Stand atop a foam roller, facing a chair with your feet parallel and pointed forward. You should be able to see the front of your feet when looking down. Keep your hands light against the chair.

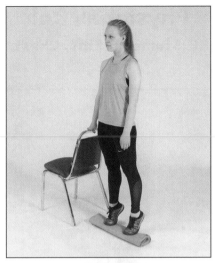

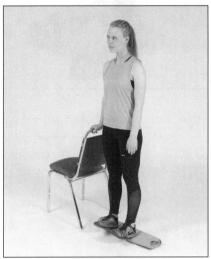

Begin by pressing the balls of your feet into the ground, then pull your heels up towards the back of your hips. To increase the effort on the calves and feet, perform the movement higher off the ground and on a single leg.

Physioball Roll

FEEL IT HERE: Stomach, Ribs, Chest, Shoulders

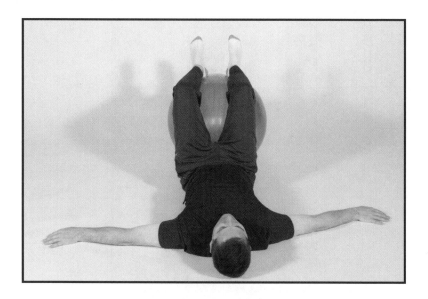

Cup your legs over a physio-ball at an angle slightly greater than 90 degrees, or a square angle at the knees and hips. Position your arms out to the side with palms down to aid in stability during lower body movement.

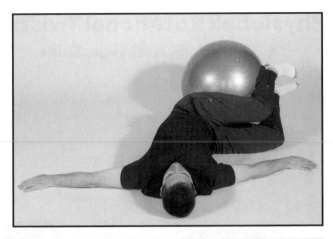

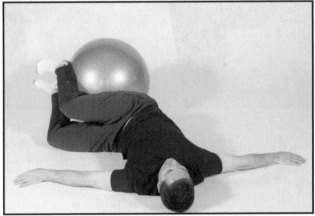

On the way toward the floor, breathe in and gently press the back of your legs into the ball thereby slowing the legs down. On the way back to your starting position, breathe out and press your hand into the floor to activate the stomach and shoulders.

Physioball Rotational Twists
FEEL IT HERE: Glutes, Legs, Spine

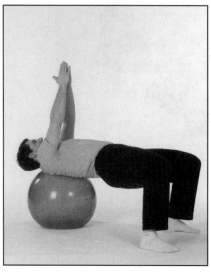 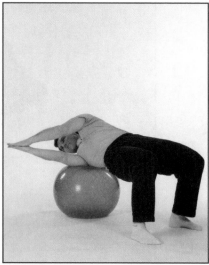

Begin sitting upright on the physioball. Keep your feet in front of your hips and "walk" to the left on the ball. Repeat to the right side. The on-back version will be completed in the same manner, but your beginning position will be on your back.

Prone Extension

FEEL IT HERE: Back, Hips

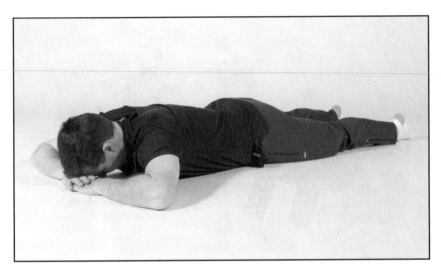

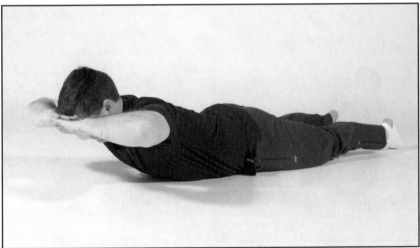

Gently press the front of your lower body into the ground. Initiate the lifting movement from your head, then shoulders, middle back, and lower back. Hold, then release slowly.

Physioball Walkup

FEEL IT HERE: Hips, Legs

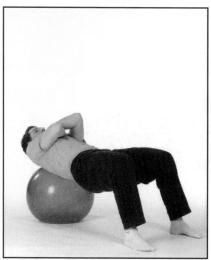

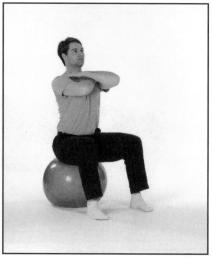

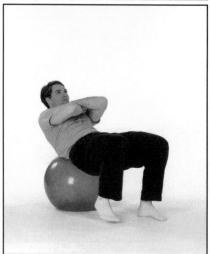

Position your hips on top of the physio-ball. Brace your core. Walk up the ball using your full foot. Keeping the feet wider adds stability if you feel off balance during the up or down phases.

Chair Stretch

FEEL IT HERE: Mid-section

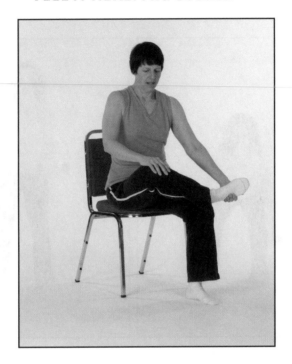

Sit upright with your hips at the same height as the knees. Breathe out and release the pressure. Pause, then assist the knees out farther. For additional support, sit against a chair back. Make sure the non-stretching hip stays firmly planted in the seat.

Curling and Pressing Combo
FEEL IT HERE: Arms, Shoulders

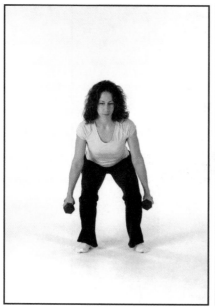 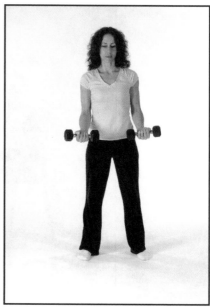

Position yourself in a half-squat position. Dumbbells should be by the sides of your body. Brace your core.

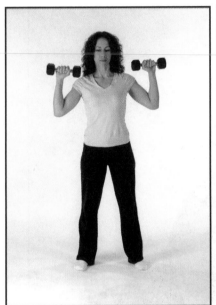 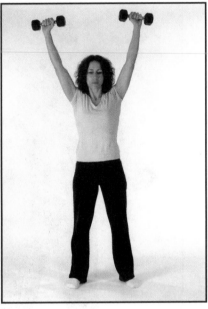

Curl the dumbbells up first and then, press them above your head, keeping your shoulders in a neutral position.

Chest Stretch (Wide Arms)
FEEL IT HERE: Chest, Shoulders, Arms

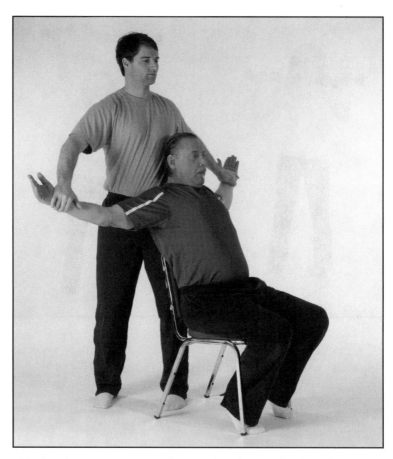

Stand behind your partner with your hands gently placed upon his or her upper arms. Keep your body positioned along your partner's spine to stabilize and assist in creating a greater stretch through the front of your partner's body.

Alphabet Series: T

FEEL IT HERE: Chest, Back

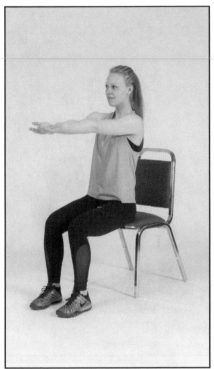 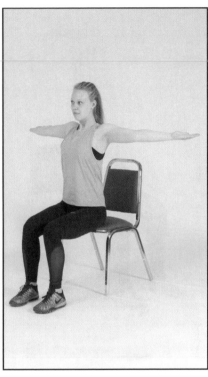

Sit upright on a sturdy surface. Squeeze your shoulder blades back and down. Draw both arms out from the mid-line of the body with palms up.

Alphabet Series: Y

FEEL IT HERE: Arms, Upper Back, Middle Back

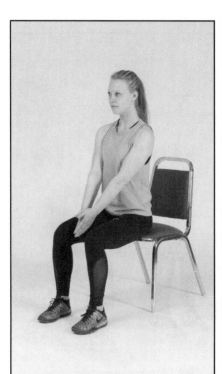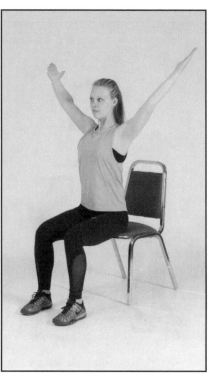

Sit upright on a sturdy surface. Squeeze your shoulder blades back and down. Draw both arms up, and straight out in front of your body at a 45-degree angle

Alphabet Series: W

FEEL IT HERE: Arms, Shoulders, Upper/Middle Back

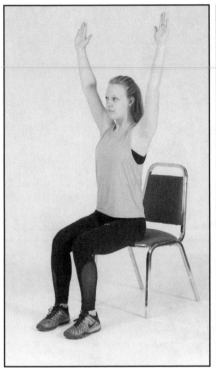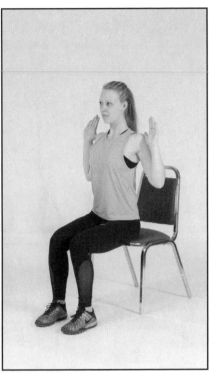

Sit upright on a sturdy surface. Squeeze your shoulder blades back and down. Draw both elbows down and back into the middle spine. Hold, then release.

Band Pull-Aparts

FEEL IT HERE: Arms, Upper Back

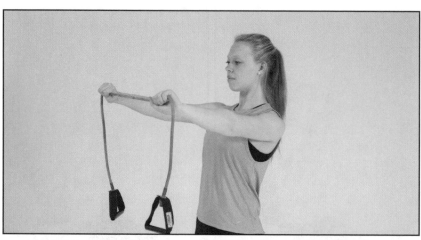

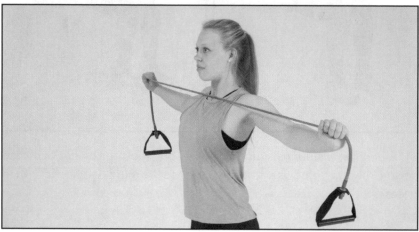

Keep the weight of your body in the feet and hips by slightly leaning forward. This allows the shoulders and arms to move naturally. Cue the shoulder blades to stay back and down thereby relaxing the upper neck muscles.

Band Pulls with One Knee Up

FEEL IT HERE: Shoulders, Arms, Hips, Legs

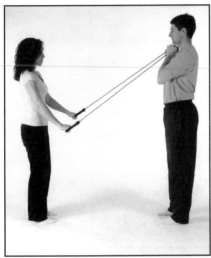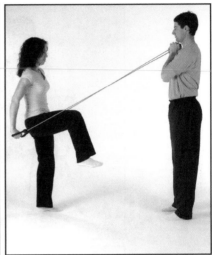

In a standing position, pull your knee upward towards your chest while pulling the arms to the sides of your body. Keep your ribs heavy and core contracted during each pressing repetition. Breathe out during each pressing rep and breathe in upon returning to the starting position.

Band Rows

FEEL IT HERE: Arms, Shoulders

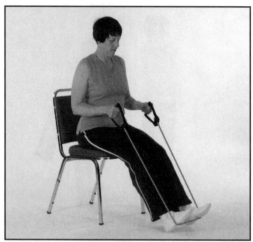

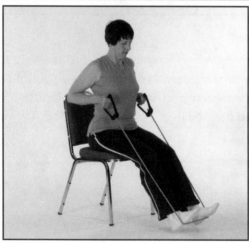

Position your body in an upright position on either a ball or bench. First, pull your shoulder blades back. Keeping them back, pull one elbow back at a time. Keep your ribs heavy and core contracted during each pressing repetition. Breathe out during each rep and breathe in upon return to the starting position. This exercise can also be done while standing.

Draw the Sword

FEEL IT HERE: Shoulder, Back

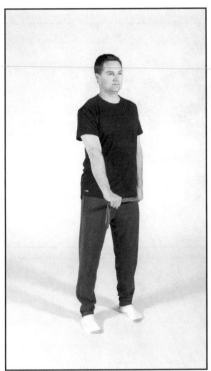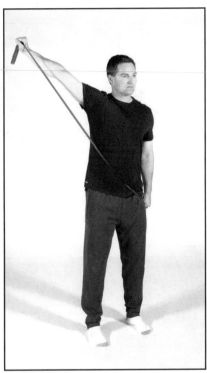

Perform this exercise sitting or standing. Reach across the body—palm down—to the opposite pocket. Imagine that you are pulling a sword and drawing it across your body. Rotate the hand and shoulder as your arm moves to the ending position, palm facing up.

Dumbbell Chest Press with Physioball

FEEL IT HERE: Chest, Shoulders, Arms

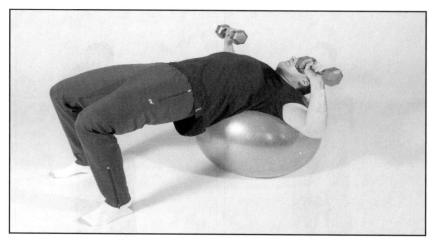

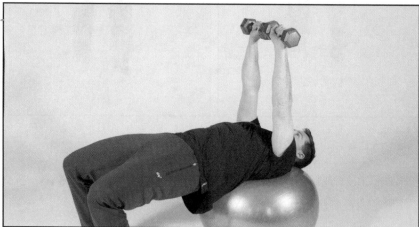

This exercise can be completed on a bench or using a physioball for an increasingly difficult exercise. Position feet slightly wider than the hips and keep feet firm on the floor. Bring the dumbbells down to a position in front of the shoulders. Push the dumbbells back up in an alternating pattern, following an outside/inside path.

Double Arm Dumbbell Row

FEEL IT HERE: Shoulders, Back, Arms

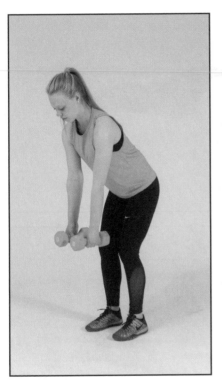 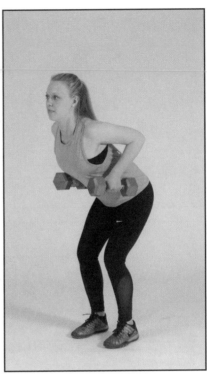

Grab a dumbbell and assume a deadlift position (lower back neutral, bent over at the waist, knees slightly bent). Place the hand without a dumbbell on your hip. Initiate the exercise by pulling your shoulder blades down and back while pulling the dumbbell up, keeping the elbow close to your body. Using only one dumbbell forces the body to use more core stability to maintain proper form.

Forward Plank

FEEL IT HERE: Stomach, Hips

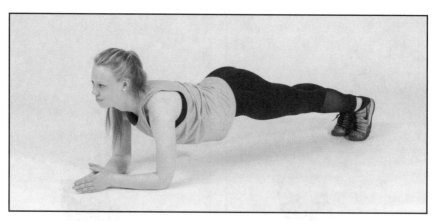

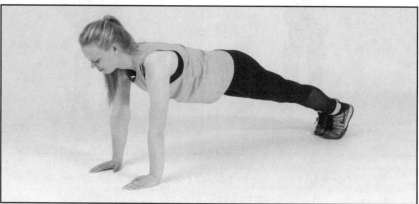

Begin on the floor, facing down. Press your palms together and your toes into the floor. Attempt to pull your upper back towards the ceiling, allowing the shoulder blades to move forward.

Lateral Plank

FEEL IT HERE: Shoulder, Mid-section, Hip

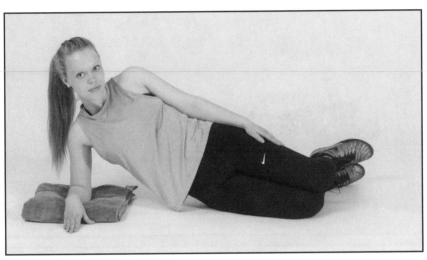

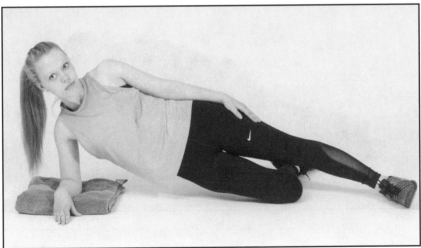

Position your body on one side, on your elbow and hip. Contract the side of your stomach and elevate your hip into alignment with the shoulders and knees.

Push-ups

FEEL IT HERE: Chest, Shoulders, Mid-section

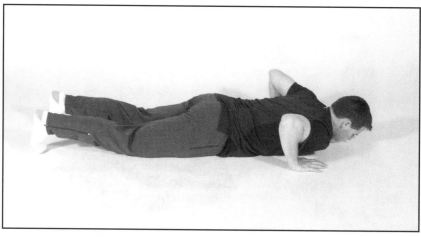

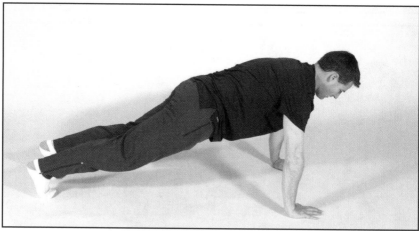

Position yourself on your stomach. Your hands should be parallel to your shoulders. Place a dowel stick along the spine so contact is made with your head and sacrum. Begin the movement by bracing your stomach. Push your toes and hands into the floor, then attempt to press your body away from the floor until your elbows are straight. You should feel your shoulder blades come together as you return to your starting position.

All-4s

FEEL IT HERE: Shoulders, Core, Legs

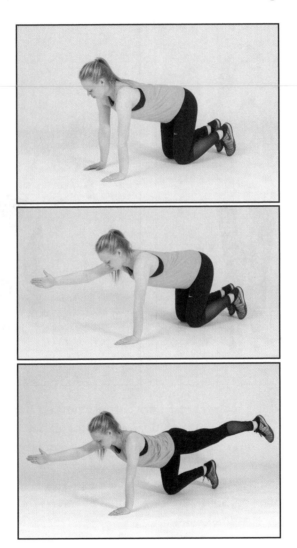

Starting on all fours, extend your opposite arm and leg, stabilizing with the hand and knee on the ground. Hold this extended position, then return to neutral.

Hip Hinging

FEEL IT HERE: Hip, Back

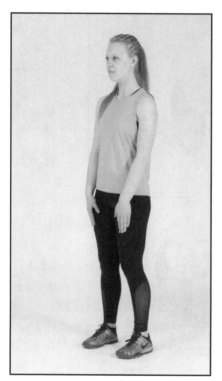 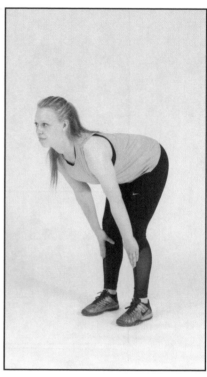

Start the squatting movement from your hips, letting the other parts follow. Feel your upper body positioned over the upper thighs as you bend during the downward motion. Brace your stomach, then begin the upward movement by pressing your feet into the floor, followed by pushing your hips through. For added help with stability, place a broomstick along your spine. Contact should be felt on the back of your head, middle back and tailbone.

Kegels

FEEL IT HERE: Pelvis, Stomach, Hips

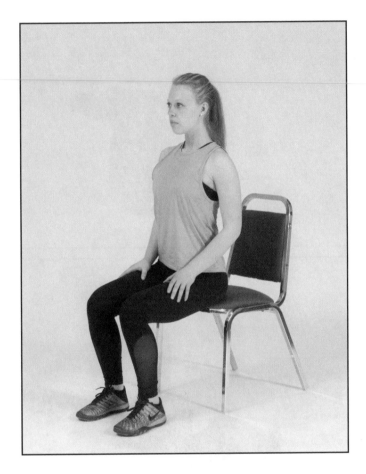

Begin by sitting on a physioball or chair. Pull your pelvic floor up and hold position.

Deadbug

FEEL IT HERE: Core

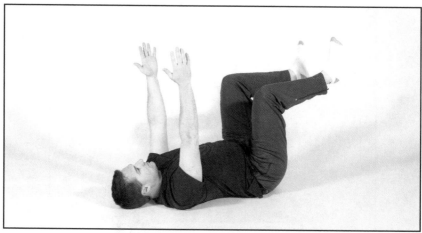

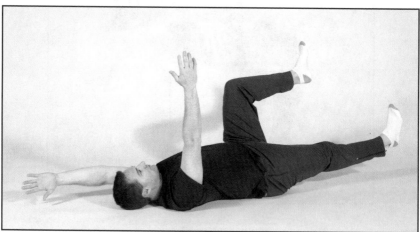

Starting on your back, begin with arms straight in front and knees bent over at the hips. Extend one arm, adding the opposite leg if you can keep your back from arching. Repeat sequence on other side.

Reverse Hyperextension
with Physioball

FEEL IT HERE: Hips, Back

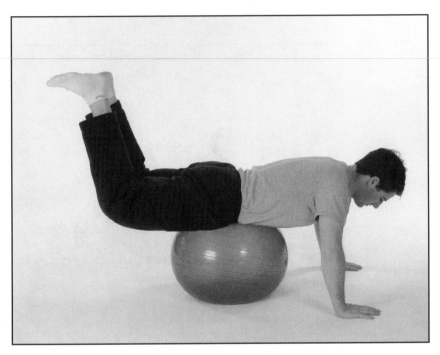

Lay on your stomach on the physioball. If you have discomfort in your neck, shoulders, or lower back, begin the exercise with one arm first. Start the movement from your middle back then lift the arm. Hold the end position. Position a pillow under your stomach/hip area for increased comfort.

Cat-Cow

FEEL IT HERE: Mid-section, Back

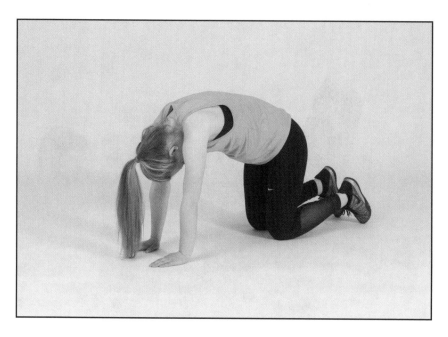

Start on your hands and knees with your wrists directly under your shoulders, and your knees directly under your hips. Place your shins and knees hip-width apart, with your head centered.

Inhale as you lower your stomach while at the same time lifting your chin and chest, and tilting your head back to look at the ceiling. This is Cow pose.

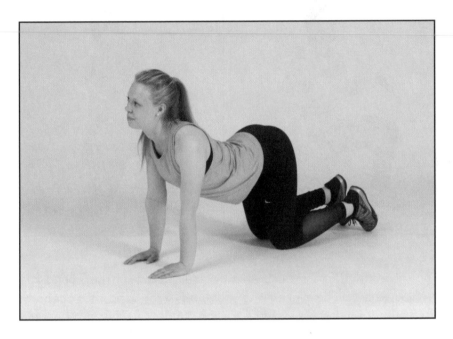

Next, move into Cat pose by exhaling and drawing your stomach to your spine. Round your back toward the ceiling. The pose should look like a cat stretching its back. Continue the movement by inhaling and coming back into Cow pose, and then exhaling as you return to Cat pose.

Lifting Movements with Band
FEEL IT HERE: Core, Hips

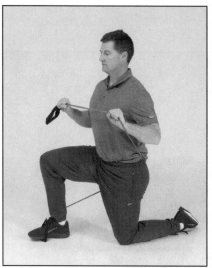 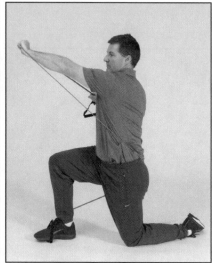

You will be lifting across your body over a trailing knee on the ground. The front knee should be aligned with your hip. Pull the band into your body, then push it up and out with the trailing hand. Keep your spine neutral by concentrating on bracing your stomach and stabilizing the hips. Think about moving around a stable pillar in your spine.

Back to Back Butterfly Stretch
FEEL IT HERE: Hips, Groin

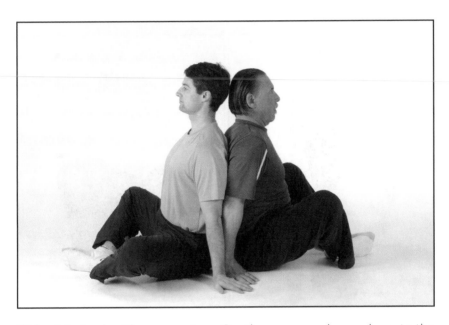

Sit back to back with your partner. Gently press your knees down to the sides, as far as they will go. Bring your core inwards, leaning forward from your hips, and grab your feet with your hands. Slowly lean forward, holding the knee position. Increase the intensity of the stretch by pressing your thighs further into the floor while holding position.

Straight Leg Deadlift

FEEL IT HERE: Legs, Hips, Mid-section

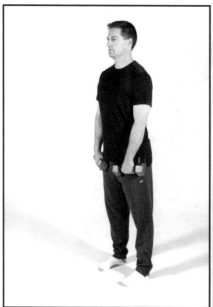 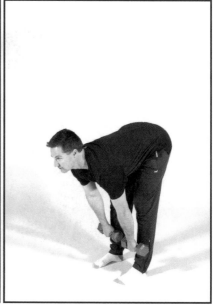

With your feet hip to shoulder-width apart and arms extended downward grabbing the barbell or dumbbell, press your feet into the floor, brace your stomach, and begin the upward ascent. Breathe out on the exertion or upward movement, pausing at the top. Begin the downward movement with the hips first, showing the chest forward.

Single Leg Deadlift

FEEL IT HERE: Legs, Hips

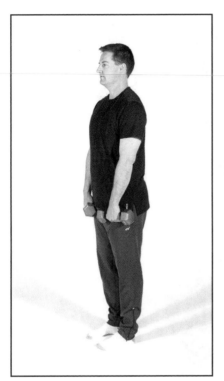 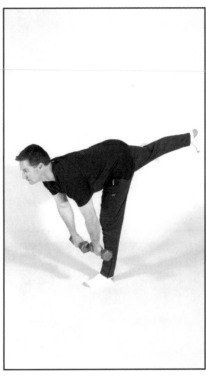

Standing up tall on one leg, place your hands on your hips and slightly bend your knees. Initiate the exercise by only moving your hips back while keeping your chest up. Initiate the exercise by kicking your balance leg back until you feel a good stretch in the hamstring of the leg on the floor. You may use an anchor point for your hands if you are having trouble balancing or if you want to emphasize stretching over balance. This variation of the movement places additional focus on the hamstrings.

Foot Taps

FEEL IT HERE: Shins

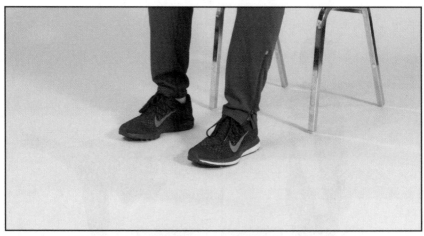

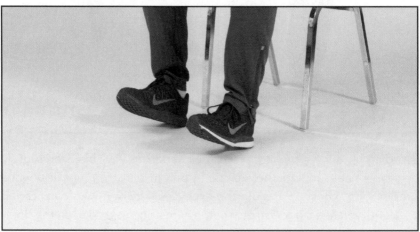

Begin in a sitting position towards the end of a chair. Tap your toes up and down together as quickly as possible, keeping your heels on the floor.

Forward Lunge

FEEL IT HERE: Hips, Legs

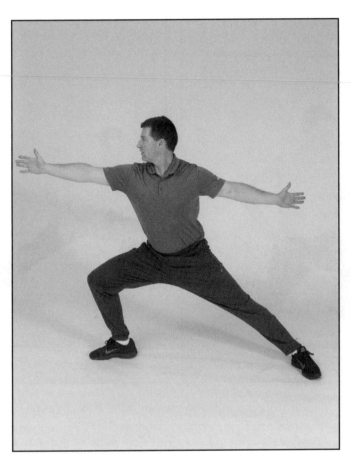

Stand with feet hip-width apart. Step forward with your right leg, shifting your weight forward so your heel hits the floor first. Lower your body until your right thigh is parallel to the floor and right shin is vertical. If mobility allows, lightly tap your left knee to the floor while keeping your weight on the right heel. Press into the right heel to drive back up to the starting position.

Clock Lunge

FEEL IT HERE: Legs, Hips

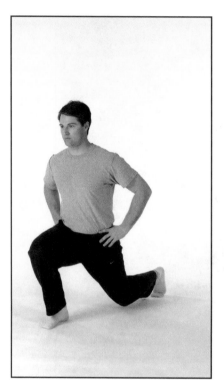 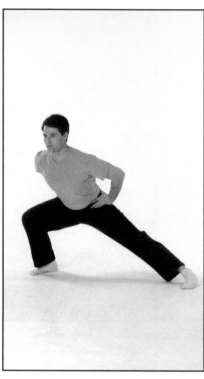

Imagine you are standing in the middle of a clock face. Lunge to various positions on the clock face. Lunging needs to be executed with proper movement at the hip and knee. Sit the hips down and back into each number on the clock face.

Stationary Lunge/Split Squat
FEEL IT HERE: Hips, Legs

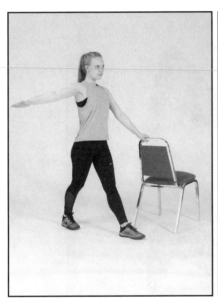 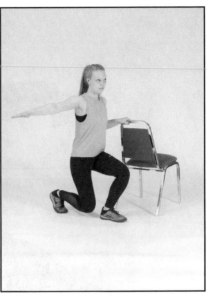

Assume a half-kneeling position with your right knee down and left knee up. Keeping your chest up and your shoulder blades pulled down and back (as though you were trying to put your shoulder blades into your back pocket), initiate the exercise by driving your left heel into the ground to push your hips up until your left leg is fully extended. Finish the movement by bending your left knee to lower yourself into a squatting position, until your right knee lightly taps the floor. You may hold onto an anchor point for balance, if needed.

Glute Bridge

FEEL IT HERE: Legs, Hips, Back

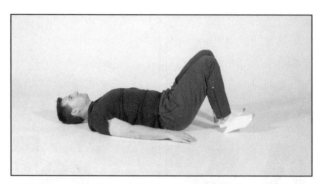

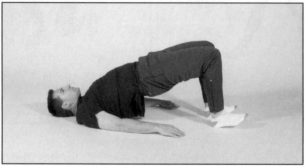

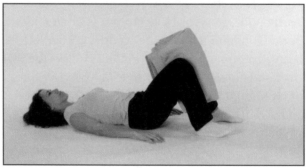

Lying supine with your knees bent and feet flat on the floor, contract your glutes and raise your hips off the floor until your body is in a straight line. Perform 1–3 sets of 10–15 repetitions.

Progress to a Single Leg Hip Bridge, then to performing the bridging action with feet on a physio/stability ball.

Windshield Wiper

FEEL IT HERE: Hips

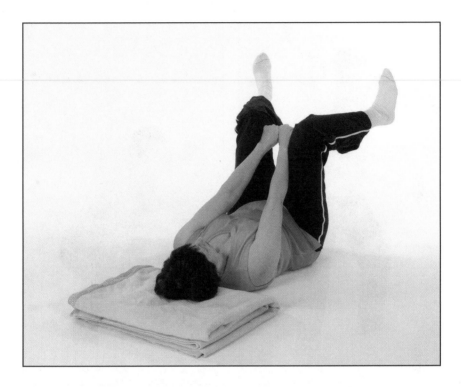

Lie on your back and raise your legs 90 degrees. With your arms spread out to your sides for support, rotate your legs to one side, stopping just short of touching the floor. Rotate to the other side for one full rep.

Open Hip Squat
FEEL IT HERE: Hips, Legs

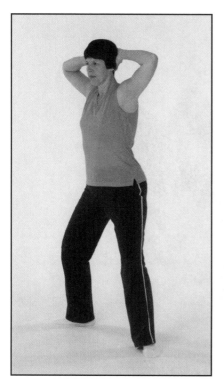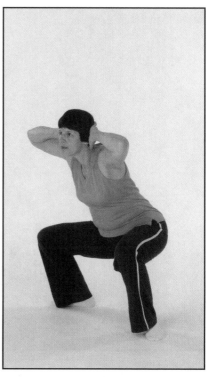

Begin by standing in a neutral stance. Your hands can be across/in front of your shoulders or behind your head. Visualizing a clock face, step away from the midline of your body, opening your hip stance to 12 and 3 o'clock (stepping to the left) or 12 and 9 o' clock (stepping to right). Once in this open stance, drop your hips into a squat. Feel the stretch in the groin and hips. This open hip squat will enhance activation of the glutes.

Spiderman

FEEL IT HERE: Legs, Hips, Shoulders, Core

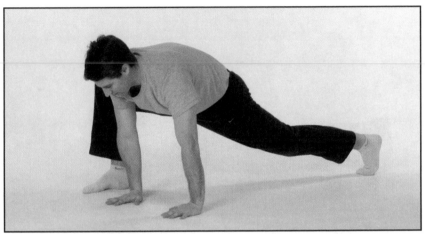

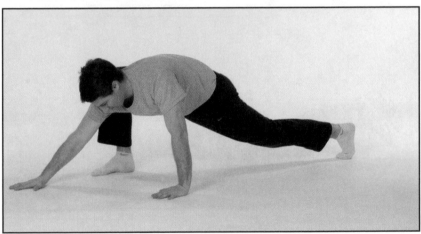

Assume a lunging position. Allow the opposite side hand to come forward with the opposite side foot. Gently rock back and forth before repeating the movement on the other side.

Supermans

FEEL IT HERE: Back, Legs

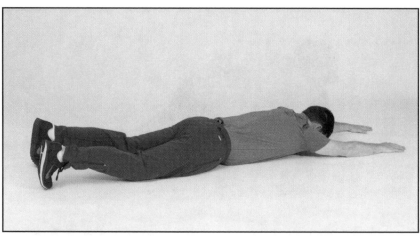

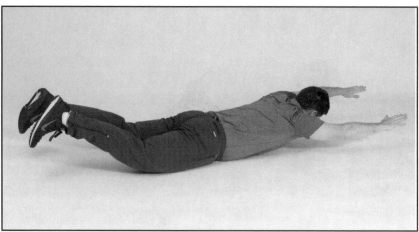

Starting on your stomach, extend your upper body off the ground. Hold this position, then return to the starting position. If you can complete this while maintaining control, repeat the sequence by lifting the upper body and legs off the ground.

Wall Sit with Foam Roller

FEEL IT HERE: Legs, Hips

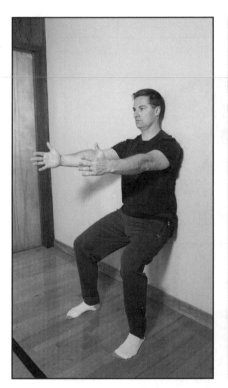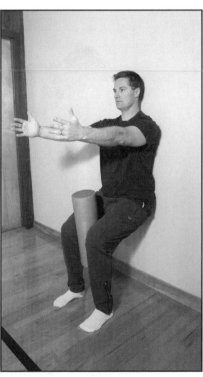

With your feet and knees hip-width apart, squeeze the foam roller between the knees. Keep your hips and shoulders against a wall. Hold the position.

Doggy Door
FEEL IT HERE: Hips, Core

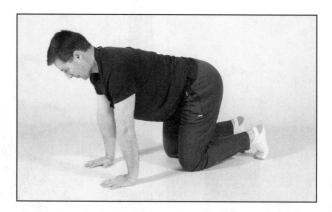

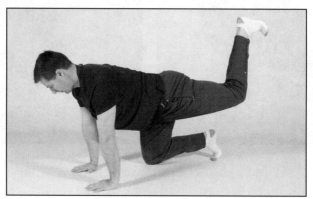

Position yourself on your hands and knees with your hands directly below your shoulders and knees directly under your hips. Your torso should be parallel to the floor with the low back flat in a neutral lumbar spine. Perform a small circle with your knee, maintaining this position.

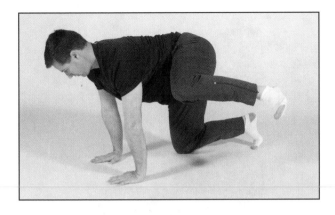

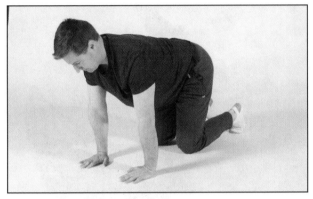

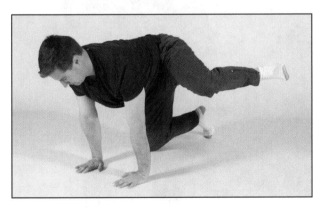

Gradually increase the size of the circle while maintaining the starting position. Perform 10–15 repetitions and then reverse the direction of the circle. Repeat on both sides for 1–3 sets.

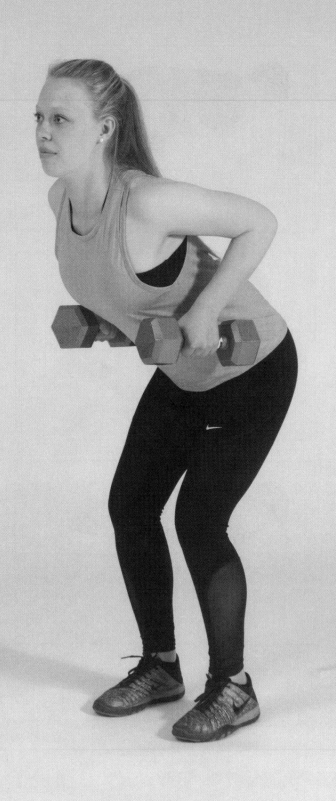

CHAPTER 7

Exercise Programs and Progressions

Everyone reading this book is at a different point in their journey towards a life free of sciatic pain. You may have just recently been cleared for exercise, or you may have an existing routine already and are looking to supplement your current program; perhaps you're exploring new approaches to manage your sciatica.

For this reason, *Exercises for Sciatica* has been designed to offer options for:
- Phasing in a new exercise program
- Replacing parts of current program
- Adding specific exercises to your current program

PROGRAM OVERVIEW
The programs outlined in this book follow a systematic approach to progress you from potentially a low level of total work capacity to one that meets the needs of your activities of improved daily living. The following are the most up-to-date exercise guidelines, intended as recommendations for individuals with sciatica:

GENERAL GUIDELINES

	LEARNING PROGRAMS: THE BASICS	TRANSITIONAL PROGRAMS: FOCUSED HACKS	GENERAL HEALTH PROGRAMS	REASSESSMENT
Cycle	2–4 weeks	4 weeks Pick 2–3 based on Assessment results (page 128)	8 weeks	4 months Repeat Assessments (page 128)
Frequency	4–5days/week	2 non-consecutive days per week of work on areas needing improvement as identified in the Assessments.	Minimum of 3 days per week, preferably 4 or more days per week.	
Intensity	RPE of 3–5 out of 10 RPE scale.	Perform 45 seconds; RPE of 6 out of 10 RPE scale.	Perform 60 seconds; RPE of 7 out of 10 RPE scale.	
Time	30 minutes total work time; 3 sets of 15 reps or 30–40 seconds/set	45 minutes total work time 3 sets of 15 reps per movement	45 minutes total work time 3–4 sets of 12 reps	
Type	Various forms may be used, but primarily body weight and bands.	Various forms may be used, not limited to body weight, bands, dumbbells.	Various forms may be used, including but not limited to body weight, bands, dumbbells.	

Aerobic Exercise Guidelines

While we often classify this area of an exercise prescription as aerobic, a better term may be cardiovascular, as it encompasses all three systems of energy development. Since each of these systems play a critical role in how we perform on a daily basis, it only makes sense that an exercise program will incorporate all three.

	FREQUENCY	INTENSITY	TIME	TYPE
Aerobic	Minimum of 2–3 non-consecutive days per week, preferably 3 or more	40–80 percent of exercise capacity. RPE of 12–16 on a scale of 6–20.	Begin with 5–10 minutes steady state movement; build up to 20–30 minutes. If too difficult, break up into 2–3 segments of 10 minutes.	Various forms may be used, including rower, treadmill, bike, elliptical.

PROGRAM VARIABLES	TRANSITION WEEK	LEVEL 1	LEVEL 2	LEVEL 3
Duration	3–5 days	2–4 weeks	5–10 weeks	2–4 weeks
Sets per exercise	–	1–3	≥ 3	≥ 3
Reps per set	–	12–15	10–12	6–12
Rest between sets	–	30 seconds	30–60 seconds	30–90 seconds

Strength Training

Resistance training is an important component to any fitness program. This becomes even more evident when recovery is the focus. Not only does resistance training provide a stimulus to the cardiovascular system, it also increases our economy of movement, meaning that we become more efficient with our normal daily tasks or ADLs. Think about this way: if we increase our levels of muscular fitness (i.e. strength and endurance), everything we do becomes easier and thereby places less stress on the body.

Multi-Joint Movements

When designing a resistance training program, including compound multi-joint movements that work the major muscle groups of the body is a must. This includes exercises like squats, lunges, step-ups, and upper body pushing and pulling, just to name few. We also include some single joint isolation exercises where appropriate. This is not only a time-efficient way to train, but also places the most demand on and creates the most stimulus for the body creating a better response per workout. These exercises are also considered more functional in nature and have a better carry-over to everyday life.

We employ many of the same principles seen in traditional aerobic fitness, using a progressive program that adds both volume and intensity over the course of several weeks. This allows for sufficient time to adapt to the new training stimulus. Unlike cardiovascular training, the frequency will be much less, based on the fact that more recovery is needed between sessions to allow the muscles involved to repair and regenerate, thereby getting stronger. Too much volume or frequency in the beginning will not allow you to have sufficient recovery between sessions.

As you become familiar with the exercises, you may begin to systematically swap out exercises for other, biomechanically similar ones.

The Complete Sciatica Recovery and Healthy Living Program

PROGRAMS

Introductory

- Complete Mobility, Physical Assessments, and Activities of Daily Living
- Complete Learning Program, Focus Points, Transitional Program and General Health progressions

Beginning the Program

Using the results of your assessments, determine which of the following areas to concentrate on. Remember to select routines based upon those areas needing improvement and your personal preference.

Upper Body. While it may seem strange to feature upper body workouts in a book on sciatica recovery, you have to learn to look at the body as one integrated system. What the upper body does, the lower body follows, and vice versa. Exercises to the upper body allow for better use of the midsection and lower body.

Midsection. The midsection, commonly known as the core, connects the upper and lower body and, from a functional perspective, the hip girdle. Many of the major organs, muscles, large swaths of connective tissue, spine, and pelvic floor are found in this area. Research indicates that the body first moves in this area when properly initiating secondary action in the arms and legs. For people with recurrent back pain, low grade inflammation tends to linger here, shutting down the primary muscles that keep the hips strong and stable.

Lower Body. The lower body includes the legs, knees, and ankles, and is our primary target area for sciatic recovery.

LEARNING THE BASICS

These are brief routines meant to slowly introduce body awareness and consistency, and integrate new activities into your daily routine. If you are currently not performing any physical activity, incorporating daily workouts may be challenge enough, and that's fine! If you are currently exercising, consider these routines as a warm-up to be done at the gym or in your home.

Introduction: Begin a Daily Habit

To start off, try one of the following (depending on when you have the most available time to exercise):
- Workout A (Morning)
- Workout B (Afternoon/Evening)

Beginner: Level I (2–4 Week Program)

General Movement Preparation
- Workout A - Focus: Upper Body

Lower Body Hack: Flexibility
- Start Workout A or Workout B

RE-ASSESS

Intermediate: Level II (6 Week Program)
Pick a workout from each of the following categories (based on your assessment). Continue with your selected workouts for two weeks each, alternating days, for 6 weeks total.

Upper Body: Flexibility
- Start Workout A or Workout B

General Movement Preparation
- Workout C - Focus: Lower Body

After 2 weeks, move on to:

Upper Body Hack: Strength
- Start Workout A or Workout B

General Movement Preparation
- Workout A - Focus: Upper Body

After another 2 weeks, move on to:

Lower Body Hack: Strength
- Start Workout A or Workout B

General Movement Preparation
- Focus: Midsection. Workout B

RE-ASSESS

Advanced: Level III (4 Week Program)

Transition Programs
- Upper Body Transition Workout A: General Health or Upper Body Transition Workout B: General Health
- Lower Body Transition Workout A: General Health or Lower Body Transition Workout B: General Health

Integrated Full Body Workouts (3 Week Program)

Start progression Workout A
- Morning Workout or Afternoon Workout

Start progression Workout B
- Morning Workout or Afternoon Workout

Start progression Workout C
- Morning Workout or Afternoon Workout

Transition Workouts (2 Week Program)

To provide your body a chance to recover from the previous workout programs, rotate back to the Learning Program routines for two weeks, then re-assess.

PROGRESSIONS

Warm-up/warm-down refers to the number of minutes that should be taken to warm-up your body before a set of exercises and the time to warm-down your body. For example, 3/3 means that you should take 4 minutes to warm-up and 4 minutes to warm-down. Rest refers to the time taken between each set of exercises. RPE refers to Rate of Perceived Exertion (see page 48 for details).

ASSESSMENTS

Based upon the outcome of the following assessments, recommendations can be made for where your focus should be during your workouts. These assessments are based on the general principles of the joint-by-joint theory, a movement approach popularized by leaders in the strength and conditioning field.

This approach focuses on the major movement centers of the body, including:
- Shoulder girdle
- Hip girdle
- Ankle complex

These three areas use various combinations of mobility and stability to execute your activities of daily living. For example, if you had a rotator cuff tear, this would create instability in your shoulder girdle, which would then affect your walking pattern: the shoulder tends to roll forward to create stability, thereby causing more torsion at the lower back and hips.

Here's another example: in the case of the lower body, if you have arthritis in your big toe, your body creates subtle adjustments in your gait by rotating your foot out or walking on the outside of the foot. This altered gait has a direct effect on your hips and lower back.

By offering an initial assessment using mobility, physical strength, and the activities of daily living as benchmarks, then scoring against a broad, simple baseline, you can re-assess using easily accessible, low-cost methods to determine areas needing improvement.

MOBILITY ASSESSMENT

Complete each assessment one time. Note any discomfort or difficulty you experience. In the third column, please rate your level of discomfort on a scale of 0–3. A score of 0 indicates pain severe enough to prohibit performing the movement. A score of 1 indicates pain which allows you to attempt, but not complete, the movement. A score of 2 indicates that you were able to complete the movement, but not without difficulty. Finally, a score of 3 indicates your ability to complete the movement without difficulty.

MOBILITY ASSESSMENT	ANY DISCOMFORT?	DISCOMFORT LEVEL
Chair Stretch		
All-4s		
Deadbug		
Overhead Squat (Hands on Wall)		
Multi-Directional Lunging Forward Lateral Reverse		
Single Leg Balancing Raise knee up with toe		

Sub-total: ——————

PHYSICAL FITNESS ASSESSMENT

PHYSICAL FITNESS ASSESSMENT	ANY DISCOMFORT?	DISCOMFORT LEVEL
Chair Stretch		
Overhead Squat with Foam Roller		
Cobra	Feel/observe any pain in the lower back. This indicates to avoid a range of motion beyond neutral, particularly if such movement has not been recently cleared by a medical professional.	
Push-ups		
Wall Sit with Foam Roller		
Supermans		
Glute Bridge		
Stationary Lunge		
Lateral Plank		

Sub-total: _____

ACTIVITIES OF DAILY LIVING ASSESSMENT

ADL ASSESSMENT	ANY DISCOMFORT?	DISCOMFORT LEVEL
Sitting		
Standing		
Walking		
Bending Over		
Driving		
Getting Up/Down		

Sub-total: _____

Total Movement Quality Score: _____

- What assessment section did you score the lowest?
- Do you see recurrent themes to focus your physical regiment?
- Pick your exercise regimen based on interest and assessment scoring
- Re-assess every 4 months

After completing each of the assessments, determine where you may want to focus your attention. Note that if you experience pain—particularly any sharp, shooting, pain—that doesn't go away, it's highly recommended that you consult with your primary care provider.

Learning Program: The Basics

FOCUS: LEARNING BASICS A

Reps: 12–15 • **Sets:** 1–2 • **Rate of Perceived Exertion:** 2–4/10
Establishes body awareness utilizing the most stable position with the largest base of support.

EXERCISE	PAGE #	EQUIPMENT/NOTES
Hip Hinging	98	
Ribs Heavy	67	
Cat-Cow	102	Limit range of motion if any irritation in back/hip
All-4s	97	
Glute Bridge with Towel	112	Towel

FOCUS: LEARNING BASICS B

Reps: 10–12 • **Sets:** 1–2 • **Rate of Perceived Exertion:** 5/10

Advancing from ground-based to standing movements, integrating major movement areas (shoulder girdle, hip girdle and ankle complex) while progressively decreasing base of support.

EXERCISE	PAGE #	EQUIPMENT/NOTES
Shoulder Circles	72	Foam roller
Thoracic Flex	61	Foam roller
Glute Bridge with Band Around Knees	112	If discomfort exists in hip/back, don't use band. Substitute towel between knees or lateral plank.
Hip Hinging	98	
Squat with Reach Across	73	Body weight

General Movement Preparation

FOCUS: GENERAL MOVEMENT PREPARATION A: UPPER BODY

Reps: 10–12 • **Sets:** 2 • **Rate of Perceived Exertion:** 5/10

Goal: To enhance upper body alignment and awareness through strengthening and mobility exercises.

EXERCISE	PAGE #	EQUIPMENT/NOTES
Shoulder Circles	72	Foam roller
Thoracic Flex	61	Foam roller
Ribcage Opener	66	Foam roller or folded towel
Alphabet Series: Y	86	Body weight optional with chair
Alphabet Series: T	85	Body weight optional with chair

FOCUS: GENERAL MOVEMENT PREPARATION B: MIDSECTION

Reps: 12–15 • **Sets:** 3 • **Rate of Perceived Exertion:** 6/10

EXERCISE	PAGE #	EQUIPMENT/NOTES
Cranial Release	62	Foam roller
Deadbug	100	Roller or floor
Ribcage Opener	66	Body weight with towel as cue
Band Pull-Aparts	88	Band
Squat with Reach Across	73	Physioball

FOCUS: GENERAL MOVEMENT PREPARATION C: LOWER BODY

Reps: 12-15 • **Sets:** 3 • **Rate of Perceived Exertion:** 6/10

Goal: To enhance lower body stability and mobility through exercises that focus on pliability, flexibility, and integrative movement patterns.

EXERCISE	PAGE #	EQUIPMENT/NOTES
Glute Roller	60	Foam roller
Scissor Stretch with Roller	68	Foam roller
Quad Roller	59	Foam roller
Physioball Walkup	80	Physioball
Open Hip Squat	114	

FOCUS: CORE WORKOUT A

Reps: 10-12 • **Sets:** • **Rate of Perceived Exertion:** 5/10

Goal: To enhance lower body stability and mobility through exercises that focus on pliability, flexibility, and integrative movement patterns.

EXERCISE	PAGE #	EQUIPMENT/NOTES
Kegels	99	Chair or physioball
Physioball Roll	76	Physioball
Forward Plank	94	Cue to pull shoulder blades forward; straighten arms to modify exercise
Lateral Plank	95	Showing bent knee, extend bottom knee to increase difficulty
Prone Extension	79	Body weight

FOCUS: CORE WORKOUT B

Reps: 12-15 • **Sets:** 3 • **Rate of Perceived Exertion:** 6/10

Goal: To establish stability in the mid-section with local and coordinated body movements.

EXERCISE	PAGE #	EQUIPMENT/NOTES
Thoracic Flex	61	Foam roller
All-4s	97	
Deadbug	100	
Lifting Band Across	104	Band
Alphabet Series: W	87	Chair

FLEXIBILITY WORKOUT A

Reps: 10-12 • **Sets:** • **Rate of Perceived Exertion:** 5/10

Goal: To enhance flexibility in areas above and below the lower spine, where sciatica often resonates.

EXERCISE	PAGE #	EQUIPMENT/NOTES
Scissor Stretch	68	Foam roller
Thoracic Flex	61	Foam roller
Chest Stretch (Wide Arms)	84	
Lateral Side Bend	-	
Back to Back Butterfly Stretch	105	Partner or wall

EXERCISE PROGRAMS AND PROGRESSIONS

FOCUS: FLEXIBILITY WORKOUT B

Reps: 12–15 • **Sets:** 3 • **Rate of Perceived Exertion:** 6/10

Goal: To enhance flexibility in areas above and below the lower spine, where sciatica often resonates, with more active movements using primary movement areas such as the hips.

EXERCISE	PAGE #	EQUIPMENT/NOTES
Straight Leg Hamstring Stretch	65	
Quad Roller	59	Foam roller
Cobra	-	Foam roller
Doggy Door	70	
Knee to Forehead	63	Body weight; single or double knee
Spiderman (Optional)	115	Body weight; advanced movement

FOCUS: GENERAL MOBILITY WORKOUT

Reps: 6-10 • **Sets:** 3 • **Rate of Perceived Exertion:** 7/10

Goal: To enhance overall movement quality with progressively more difficulty exercises that combine flexibility, strength, and self-massage techniques.

EXERCISE	PAGE #	EQUIPMENT/NOTES
Glute Bridge	112	
Hip Hinging	98	
Open Hip Squat	114	
Clock Lunge	110	
Glute Roller	60	Foam roller

FOCUS: UPPER BODY STRENGTH WORKOUT A

Reps: 10-12 • **Sets:** 3 • **Rate of Perceived Exertion:** 5/10

Goal: To enhance strength in upper body.

EXERCISE	PAGE #	EQUIPMENT/NOTES
Shoulder Circles	72	Foam roller
Push-ups	96	Body Weight
Band Rows	90	Band

FOCUS: UPPER BODY STRENGTH WORKOUT B

Reps: 6-10 • **Sets:** 3-4 • **Rate of Perceived Exertion:** 7/10

Goal: To enhance overall strength with complementary self-treatment exercises.

EXERCISE	PAGE #	EQUIPMENT/NOTES
Cranial Release	62	
Double Arm Dumbbell Row	93	Dumbbell
Draw the Sword	91	Band

FOCUS: LOWER BODY STRENGTH WORKOUT A

Reps: 6–12 • **Sets:** 3–4 • **Rate of Perceived Exertion:** 7/10

Goal: To improve lower body strength in the hips and legs, with particular focus on hip strength.

EXERCISE	PAGE #	EQUIPMENT/NOTES
Glute Bridge	112	Body weight or squeeze ball/towel between knees
Windshield Wiper	113	Body weight
Single Leg Hamstring Stretch	70	Body weight
Wall Sit with Foam Roller	117	Foam roller
Open Hip Squat	114	Body weight

FOCUS: LOWER BODY STRENGTH WORKOUT B

Reps: 6–12 • **Sets:** 3–4 • **Rate of Perceived Exertion:** 7/10

Goal: To improve lower body strength in the hips and legs, re-visiting the proper relationship between the upper and lower body, and soft-tissue treatment.

EXERCISE	PAGE #	EQUIPMENT/NOTES
Hip Hinging	98	
Gastroc Roller	58	Roller
Open Hip Squat	114	
Single Leg Deadlift	107	Dumbbell (optional)
Calf Raise/Shin Raise	74	

Transitional Workouts

TRANSITIONAL WORKOUT A

Reps: 12 • **Sets:** 2 • **Rat of Perceived Exertion:** 5/10

Goal: To improve the relationship between upper and lower body movements.

EXERCISE	PAGE #	EQUIPMENT/NOTES
All-4s	97	
Push-ups	96	
Double Arm Dumbbell Row	93	Dumbbell(s)
Open Hip Squat	114	

TRANSITIONAL WORKOUT B

Reps: 10 • **Sets:** 3 • **Rate of Perceived Exertion:** 6/10

Goal: To focus on upper and lower body strength, transitioning to integrated program section.

EXERCISE	PAGE #	EQUIPMENT/NOTES
Prayer Pose	64	Body Weight
Dumbbell Chest Press with Physioball	92	Physioball, dumbbell
Band Rows	90	Band
Band Pull-Aparts	88	Band
Stationary Lunge	111	

TRANSITIONAL WORKOUT C

Reps: 15 • Sets: 3 • Rate of Perceived Exertion: 6/10

Goal: To improve the relationship between your upper and lower body with larger, more complex movements.

EXERCISE	PAGE #	EQUIPMENT/NOTES
Double Arm Dumbbell Row	93	Use band if preferred
Shoulder Circles	72	Dumbbell
Push-ups	96	
Clock Lunge	110	
Forward Plank	94	

FOCUS: MULTITASKING INTEGRATED WORKOUT A

Reps: 12 • Sets: 4 • Rate of Perceived Exertion: 7/10

Goal: To improve overall work capacity through large muscle movements and increased volume.

EXERCISE	PAGE #	EQUIPMENT/NOTES
Quad Roller	59	Foam roller
Thoracic Flex	61	
Clock Lunge	110	Body weight
Open Hip Squat	114	
Double Arm Dumbbell Row	93	Dumbbell(s)
Dumbbell Chest Press with Physioball OR Push-ups	92,96	Dumbbell(s) or body weight

FOCUS: MULTITASKING INTEGRATED WORKOUT B

Reps: 10 • **Sets:** 4 • **Rate of Perceived Exertion:** 8/10

EXERCISE	PAGE #	EQUIPMENT/NOTES
Shoulder Circles	72	Foam roller
Glute Roller	60	Foam roller
Cat-Cow	102	
Push-ups	95	
Lateral Plank	121	
Stationary Lunges	–	
Physioball Rotational Twists	78	Physioball

FOCUS: MULTITASKING INTEGRATED WORKOUT C

Reps: 15 • **Sets:** 4 • **Rate of Perceived Exertion:** 8/10

Goal: To improve overall work capacity through large muscle movements and increased volume with new exercise combinations.

EXERCISE	PAGE #	EQUIPMENT/NOTES
Spiderman	115	
Scissor Stretch	68	Foam roller
Straight Leg Deadlift	106	Dumbbell(s)
Physioball Walkup	80	
Curl and Press	-	
Push-ups	96	Dumbbell(s)
Band Pulls with One Knee Up	88	Band

PREPARING FOR A DOCTOR'S APPOINTMENT

Not everyone who has sciatica needs medical care. However, if your symptoms are severe or persist for more than a month, make an appointment with your primary care doctor.

The following are some basic guidelines to help you prepare for your appointment, to make sure that everyone involved has all the information needed to make accurate recommendations. Of course, you shouldn't hesitate to ask any other questions you might have, but these are meant to provide tips for those seeking treatment for back and sciatic nerve pain.

What you can do to prepare:
- Write down your symptoms and when they began.
- List key medical information, including other conditions you have and the names of medications, vitamins or supplements you take.
- Note any recent accidents or injuries that might have damaged your back.
- Take a family member or friend along, if possible. Someone who accompanies you can help you remember what your doctor tells you.
- Write down questions to ask your doctor to make the most of your appointment time.

For radiating low back pain, some basic questions to ask your doctor include:
- What's the most likely cause of my back pain?
- Are there other possible causes?
- Do I need diagnostic tests?
- What treatment do you recommend?
- If you're recommending medications, what are the possible side effects?
- For how long will I need to take medication?

- Am I a candidate for surgery? Why or why not?
- Are there restrictions I need to follow?
- What self-care measures should I take?
- What can I do to prevent my symptoms from recurring?

Your doctor is also likely to ask you a number of questions, like:
- Do you have numbness or weakness in your legs?
- Do certain body positions or activities make your pain better or worse?
- How limiting is your pain?
- Do you do heavy physical work?
- Do you exercise regularly? If yes, with what types of activities?
- What treatments or self-care measures have you tried? Has anything helped?

RESOURCES

ORGANIZATIONS

American Academy of Orthopedic Surgeons

Website: www.aaos.org

Website: orthoinfo.org

Toll-Free Phone Number: (847) 823-7186

National Institute of Arthritis and Musculoskeletal and Skin Diseases

Website: www.niams.nih.gov

Toll-Free Phone Number: (877) 226-4267

SOCIAL MEDIA GROUPS

Sciatica Pain Relief Community (Facebook group)

15K members, 10+ posts a day. This group is designed to help surround you with people who understand the daily struggles associated with back pain and sciatica.

Sciatica Pain Management (Facebook page)

Described as a community interested in back pain or sciatica pain research studies, they collect information to be freely shared among community members.

Back Pain & Sciatica Sufferer Support (Facebook group)

25K members, 10+ posts a day.

Sciatica & Back Pain Awareness Forum (Facebook group)

6.4K members, 3 posts a day. Provides a safe space where people can talk about their experiences with back pain and sciatica.

BLOGS

The Sciatica Authority

www.sciatica-pain.org/sciatica-blog.html

OTHER RESOURCES

Tom Myers' Anatomy Trains

www.anatomytrains.com

This is a fabulous resource for helping people understand the inner workings of the body's muscular systems

ABOUT THE AUTHORS

William Smith, MS, CSCS, MEPD, currently works for a nationally recognized healthcare system in the New York metropolitan area providing health and wellness services to the community. His interest is in special populations and how healthcare providers and fitness professionals can work more closely together. Will completed his B.S. in exercise science followed by an MS at St. John's University where he was the Assistant Director of Strength and Conditioning. Will has been featured on NBC, Canyon Ranch, World Spinning Conference and in Homecare Magazine.

Wazim Buksh, MD, MPH is board certified in both sports medicine and internal medicine. He currently practices both specialties as the lead physician for Primary Care at Novartis, an Atlantic Health System's practice, in New Jersey. He has worked with the New York Jets and the athletic departments of Seton Hall and Drew Universities, respectively. In addition, he has provided sports coverage for a multitude of high schools in the New Jersey area. Dr. Buksh practices with a focus towards prevention—keeping you healthy to enjoy life's journey.

ALSO IN THIS SERIES

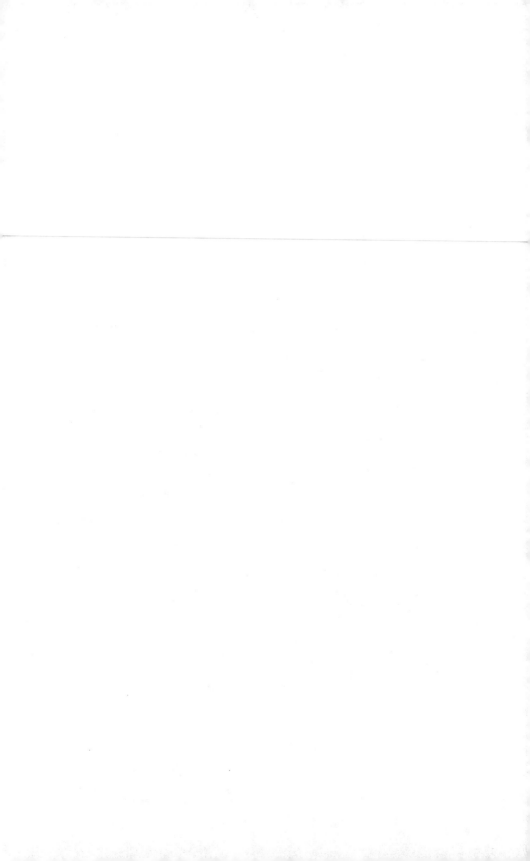